Pediatric Development and Neonatology

Christine M. Houser

Pediatric Development and Neonatology

A Practically Painless Review

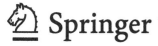 Springer

Christine M. Houser
Department of Emergency Medicine
Erasmus Medical Center
Rotterdam, The Netherlands

ISBN 978-1-4614-8680-0   ISBN 978-1-4614-8681-7 (eBook)
DOI 10.1007/978-1-4614-8681-7
Springer New York Heidelberg Dordrecht London

Library of Congress Control Number: 2013947469

Printed on acid-free paper

Springer is part of Springer Science+Business Media (www.springer.com)

To my parents Martin and Cathy who made this journey possible, to Patrick who travels with me, and to my wonderful children Tristan, Skyler, Isabelle, Castiel, and Sunderland who have patiently waited during its writing – and are also the most special of all possible reminders for why pediatric medicine is so important.

Important Notice

Medical knowledge and the accepted standards of care change frequently. Conflicts are also found regularly between various sources of recognized literature in the medical field. Every effort has been made to ensure that the information contained in this publication is as up-to-date and accurate as possible. However, the parties involved in the publication of this book and its component parts, including the author, the content reviewer, and the publisher, do not guarantee that the information provided is in every case complete, accurate, or representative of the entire body of knowledge for a topic. We recommend that all readers review the current academic medical literature for any decisions regarding patient care.

Preface

Preparing for the general pediatric board examination can be a daunting task. Returning to general pediatric studies again for a recertification exam, or a retake of the initial exam, is a lot to take on in the midst of an ongoing practice and the many other professional and personal obligations most physicians face. It is important to find strategies and materials that make the process as efficient and flexible as possible. At the same time, exam preparations can be a great opportunity to thoroughly review the many areas involved in pediatric practice, and to consolidate and refresh the knowledge developed through the years so far.

Practically Painless Pediatrics brings together the information from several major pediatric board review study guides and more review conferences than any one physician would ever have time to personally attend for review. What makes this book especially unusual is that it is designed in "bite-sized" chunks of information that can be quickly read and processed, using a question-and-answer format that helps the mind to stay active while studying. This improves the speed with which the information can be learned. The two-column design also makes it possible to easily quiz yourself or to use the book for quizzing in pairs or groups studying together. A simple Q & A format means that answers are not paragraphs long, as is often the case in medical books. Answers are quick and concise and targeted for what is needed in the board exam questions.

Because the majority of information is in Q & A format, it is also much easier to use the information in a few minutes of downtime at the hospital or office. You don't need to get deeply into the material to understand what you are reading.

For a few especially challenging topics, or for topics that can be more efficiently presented in a regular text rather than Q & A style, a text section has been provided. These sections precede the larger neonatology Q & A section. Here, neonatal physiology, in particular, is briefly discussed.

Practically Painless Pediatrics is designed for efficient studying. Very often, information provided in review books raises as many questions as it answers. This interferes with the study process, because the learner either has to look up the additional information (time loss) or skip the information entirely and therefore not really understand or learn it. This book keeps answers self-contained, meaning that any needed information is provided either in the answer, or immediately following it—all without lengthy text.

The materials utilized in *Practically Painless Pediatrics* were tested by residents and attendings preparing for the general pediatric board examination, or the recertification examination, to ensure that both the approach and content were on target. All content has also been reviewed by attending and specialist pediatricians to ensure the quality and understandability of the content.

This book utilizes the knowledge gained about learning and memory processes over many years of research into cognitive processing, to streamline the study process. All of us involved in the process of creating it sincerely hope that you will find the study process a bit less onerous with this format, and perhaps even find a bit of joy and excitement in reviewing the material!

Brief Guidance Regarding Use of the Book

Items which appear in **bold** indicate topics known to be frequent board exam content. On occasion, an item's content is known to be very specific to previous board questions. In that case, the item will have "popular exam item" beneath it.

At times, you will encounter a Q & A item that covers the same content as a previous item. These items are worded differently and often require you to process the information in a somewhat different way compared to the previous version. This variation in the way questions are asked, for the particularly challenging or important content areas, is not an error or oversight. It is designed to increase the probability that the reader will be able to retrieve the information when it is needed—regardless of how the vignette is presented on the exam or how the patient presents in a clinical setting.

Occasionally, a brand name for a medication or piece of medical equipment is included in the materials. These are always indicated with the trademark symbol (®) and are not meant to indicate an endorsement of or recommendation to use that brand name product. Brand names are occasionally included only to make processing of the study items easier, when the brand name is significantly more recognizable to most physicians than the generic name would be.

The specific word choice used in the text may at times seem informal to the reader, and occasionally a bit irreverent. Please rest assured that no disrespect is intended to anyone or any discipline in any case. The mnemonics or comments provided are only intended to make the material more memorable. The informal wording is often easier to process than the rather complex or unusual wording many of us in the medical field have become accustomed to. That is why rather straightforward wording is sometimes used, even though it may at first seem unsophisticated.

Similarly, visual space is provided on the page, so that the material is not closely crowded together. This improves the ease of using the material for self- or group quizzing, and minimizes time potentially wasted identifying which answers belong to which questions.

The reader is encouraged to use this extra space to make additional notes or comments for him or herself. Further, the Q & A format is particularly well suited to marking difficult or important items for further review and quizzing. Please consider making a system in advance to indicate which items you'd like to return to, and which items have already been repeatedly reviewed. This can also offer a handy way to know which items are most important for last-minute review—a frequently very difficult "triage" task.

Finally, consider switching back and forth between topics under review, to improve processing of new items. Trying to learn and remember too many items on similar topics at one time is often more difficult than breaking the information up by periodically switching to a different topic.

Ultimately, the most important aspect of learning the material needed for board examinations is what we as physicians can bring to our patients, and the amazing gift that patients entrust to us in letting us take an active part in their health. With that focus in mind, the task at hand is not substantially different from what each examination candidate has already done in medical school and in patient care. With that in mind, board examination studying should be both a bit less anxiety provoking and a bit more palatable. Seize the opportunity and happy studying to all!

Rotterdam, The Netherlands   Christine M. Houser

About the Author

Dr. Houser completed her medical degree at the Johns Hopkins University School of Medicine, after spending 4 years in graduate training and research in Cognitive Neuropsychology at George Washington University and The National Institutes of Health. Her Master of Philosophy degree work focused on the processes involved in learning and memory, and during this time she was a four-time recipient of training awards from The National Institutes of Health (NIH). Dr. Houser's dual interests in cognition and medicine led her naturally toward teaching and "translational cognitive science"—finding ways to apply the many years of cognitive research findings about learning and memory to how physicians and physicians-in-training might more easily learn and recall the vast quantities of information required for medical studies and practice.

Content Reviewers

For Developmental Topics:

Kim K. Cheung, MD, PhD
Assistant Professor, Department of Pediatrics,
Division of Community and General Pediatrics
University of Texas – Houston Medical School
Houston, TX, USA

For Neonatal Topics:

Suzanne M. Lopez, MD, FAAP
Associate Professor, Department of Pediatrics,
Division of Neonatal-Perinatal Medicine
University of Texas – Houston Medical School
Houston, TX, USA

Director, Division of Neonatal-Perinatal Medicine Fellowship Program
University of Texas – Houston Medical School
Houston, TX, USA

Medical Director, Neonatal Nurse Practitioners
University of Texas – Houston Medical School
Houston, TX, USA

Contents

Chapter 1
Developmental Topics

For preemies, how long should you continue to "correct" their age when evaluating developmental milestones?	Until age 2
If a child does not score well on developmental milestones, but was also uncooperative during the exam, what should you conclude?	Results are not valid
If a child does not score well on developmental milestones, but was also ill at the time of the exam, what should you conclude?	Results are not valid
In addition to a thorough history & physical examination, what else should you check in an infant with developmental delay?	The metabolic screening done by the state (sometimes abnormal results are missed)
In a preschool child with developmental delay, what two correctable reasons should always be looked for?	Hypothyroid & Lead
If a child has idiopathic mental retardation which has been present since birth, and no other signs or symptoms, should you conduct a metabolic screening?	No

C.M. Houser, *Pediatric Development and Neonatology: A Practically Painless Review*, DOI 10.1007/978-1-4614-8681-7_1, © Springer Science+Business Media New York 2014

What is the most common reason for severe mental retardation?

Down syndrome

Do mild mental retardation patients usually have chromosomal abnormalities?

No
(only about 5 %)

Which kids with mental retardation should have chromosome testing?

- Severe MR
- Family history of MR or repeated fetal losses
- Microcephalic
- Associated abnormalities

If a child has language delay, how likely is it that the child will also have delay in some other developmental areas?

Likely – 50 %

What is the usual pattern of vocalization for deaf infants?

They coo, but not interactively – no babbling

At what age should you worry about a baby that does not babble?

9 months

At what age should you worry about a baby that does not say any **words?**

18 months

When should a young child's speech be understandable to strangers most of the time?

**3 years
(Fully understandable at age 4)**

By what age should a child be able to use at least some phrases appropriately?

2 years

How long should it take for an infant to double the birth weight?

4–6 months

When 1 year old, how much should the infant weigh, compared to the birth weight?

About 3×

By what age should the birth length be doubled?

4 years

When the infant is 1 year old, how long should he/she be, compared to the birth length?

1.5×

Can tests like the "Denver Developmental" or other school screening tests diagnose learning problems?

No – they only identify kids who need more screening

Can significant language delay be normal if the child is raised in a bilingual home?

Not on the boards

If parents or siblings tend to "speak for" a child who is language delayed, can that actually cause the language delay?

No

At what age should infants be able to cruise while holding on with both hands?

10–11 months

When is pincer grasp usually well developed?

12 months

At what age do infants have a partial, inferior, pincer grasp?

10 months

If your patient can grab an object voluntarily, but cannot release the grip, what age is your patient?

5 months

At what age can children use their hand as a "rake" to gather objects?

7 months

What is the average age at which most infants will successfully play "pat-a-cake?"

**14 months
Mnemonic:
7 months "rake"
14 months "pat-a-cake"**

If the baby is lying on the belly, at what age will he/she be able to lift the head up off the floor?

2 months

At what age can the baby hold its head at 45°, if it is on its belly?	3 months
At what age can the baby hold his/her head up at 90°, when lying on the belly?	4 months
If a baby is lying on her belly, at what age can she usually push her chest up & support herself with her arms?	4 months
If you pull an infant from lying to a sitting position, at what age will the baby's head come up at the same time as the body (no head lag)?	5 months for more than 75 %, (90 % at 6 months)
At what age should infants sit *without* support?	7 months *(can sit with support at 6 months)*
Which way do infants roll first, front to back, or back to front?	**Front to back –** This is really not so hard to remember; after all, it is much easier to use your arm to push yourself onto your back
At what age will infants first roll from front to back?	**About 4 months**
How old will the infant be when he/she rolls from back to front for the first time?	**About 5 months**
Social smiling starts at what age?	1–2 months
At what age will most infants smile back at themselves, when looking in a mirror?	5 months
A child should be able to dress himself at what age?	3 years *(not including buttons or other devices in the back)*

Waving "bye-bye" usually starts at what age?	10 months
What sort of language output is expected at age 2 months?	Cooing
How far, relative to their own bodies, can 2-month-olds follow an object visually?	Past midline
At what age can your infant first put things into its mouth intentionally?	4 months
When can babies usually grab easy-to-hold objects?	4 months
At what age can infants generally transfer an object from hand to hand?	6 months
How old are most kids when they learn to jump with both feet off the ground?	2 years
At what age will most kids learn to hop on one foot?	4 years
Skipping is pretty tough. When will most kids learn to skip? (requires hopping, alternating feet, and moving forward!)	5–6 years
Which comes first, hopping or balancing on one foot for a few seconds?	Balancing for a few seconds – age 3 years
When are children able to balance on one foot for a long period of time, say 10 s?	4 years (Some say this ability is lost with age – try testing some adults!)
According to the books, when can kids tie their own shoelaces? (Warning, may not match with your personal experience, when traveling with large number of small kids!)	5 years

**What common condition will
sometimes cause the head to enlarge
rapidly in the first 6 months,
but does not require treatment?**

**Macrocephaly
(The head often grows rapidly to
its "target" size in the 6 months
following birth)**

**If rapid growth in head circumference
is occurring in the first 6 months
of life, how do you confirm that
the cause is benign?**

- **No abnormal findings on
  history/physical examination**
- **Parents also have large heads**

When do normal infants have the most
rapid growth in head circumference?

Birth – 2 months (0.5 cm/week)

How is macrocephaly defined?

Head circumference >95 %

**For preemies, should you chart
gestational age or chronological age
for head circumference?**

Gestational age

Which catches up faster for preemies,
head circumference or length & weight
growth?

Head circumference
(It can make you think preemies are
macrocephalic, when they are really
not)

Why is head circumference monitored
especially carefully in preemies?

Increased risk of hydrocephalus
(But remember that apparent
macrocephaly could be normal
catch-up growth)

**What normal variation produces
benign macrocephaly, especially
in males?**

Enlarged subarachnoid space

**If a child is born with normal
head circumference, then becomes
microcephalic, is the cause likely
to be primary or secondary?**

Secondary

**Is posterior plagiocephaly
(head flattening) usually due
to sleeping position or craniosynostosis?**

Sleeping position

If you would like to use a helmet
to decrease severe plagiocephaly,
at what age is it most useful?

0–6 months old
*(need to wear it 22 h a day to be
helpful!!!)*

How many sutures are involved in benign craniosynostosis (not associated with other problems)?

Just one –
Repair between 6 and 12 months, if needed

Until what age should stuttering be considered normal?

Roughly age 3

At what point does stuttering definitely require referral for evaluation?

School aged

At what age is a child's speech expected to be clear to anyone?

4 years
(50 % intelligible age 2)
(75 % intelligible age 3)

At what age can a child bend down to pick something up without falling over?

16 months, generally

At what age can a young child crawl into a chair on his/her own?

18 months

If an infant is developmentally normal, and he/she can build a tower of just two blocks, how old should that infant be?

About 14 months

How tall is the tower an 18-month-old builds?

Three or four blocks

At 2 years of age, how many blocks will be in the tower?

Seven

If an 18-month-old turns the pages of a book, how many will they usually turn at a time?

Three

Can a 2-year-old turn single pages in a book?

Supposedly (!)

At what age will most children be able to go up and down stairs, with both feet on each step?

2 years

When will a child be able to walk up stairs alternating feet?	**Age 3 or 4** (depends on source)
How many times should a 3-year-old be able to hop?	**Three**
At what age can a child ride a tricycle?	**Three**
How many body parts can a 4-year-old usually draw?	**Four**
At what age can most children draw a square?	**Five**
Children are usually able to pull themselves up to stand at how many months?	**9 months**
What is the average age for children to walk without help?	**12 months**
When can children walk backwards?	**Five** (**But often pull toys while walking backwards by 18 months**)
Children are good runners by about what age, on the average?	**2 years**
At what age will children be able to print letters?	**Five** (**makes sense, they start kindergarten at that point**)
What odd block task is 4-year-olds expected to be able to do?	**Build a gate of blocks**
How many colors should a 4-year-old be able to identify?	**Four**
How high should a 4-year-old be able to count?	**Four**
When can a child recite a four-word sentence?	**Age four**

At what age can children wave "bye-bye?"	**1 year**
At what age should children be good at using gestures?	**18 months**
At what age can a child use pronouns appropriately?	**3 years**
At what age can most children use plurals correctly?	**3 years**
What are the "P's" of language development at age 3 years?	**Uses: Preposition, plurals, pronouns, and short paragraphs**
At what age should most children use the past tense correctly?	**4 years**
When should children be able to tell a simple story?	**4 years** **Mnemonic:** **Remember that you might need to use the past tense to tell a story – at 4 years old, kids can both use the past tense and tell a short story!**
By what age should children have mastered tough English-language sounds like "th," "s," and "r?"	6 years
At what age can most infants drink from a cup?	50 % by 12 months
By what age are infants usually fairly good at using a spoon & cup?	18 months
When a significant family stressor, such as divorce, occurs in a preschooler's family, how will he/she usually react?	Regression (behaving like a younger child)
How do adolescents commonly react to serious family stressors, such as divorce?	**Depression & suicidal ideation**

How do early school-aged children usually react to a difficult divorce?

Grief –
Crying is common

Do older school-aged children react differently to divorce, compared to the early school-aged kids?

Yes –
More anger than grief

School-aged children often show distress due to difficult family situation with what three symptoms?

- **Sleep disturbances**
- **Declining school performance**
- **Somatization (headaches, stomach aches)**

Are disorders such as asthma, eczema, or migraine headaches "psychosomatic?"

No –
Although stress can contribute to them

How does "perceived control" of a situation affect the stress a child feels in that situation?

Generally, more perceived control means less stress
(Actual control is not as important as "perceived control")

If a child is language delayed, what is the first test you should do?

Hearing evaluation

What is the most common cause of conductive hearing loss?

Fluid in the middle ear

If a child has severe hearing loss, is that likely to be conductive or sensorineural?

Nearly always sensorineural
(high frequencies affected most)

Are most term infants nearsighted or farsighted at birth?

Nearsighted (myopic) –
Remember, that is how they are so good at focusing on faces just a few inches away from theirs while breast feeding!

Are most preemies nearsighted or farsighted?

Usually farsighted
(hyperopic)

Are learning differences (aka learning disabilities) related to the intelligence of the child?

Not really –
A learning difference means that there is a significant impairment in one aspect of cognition, compared to the others

Generally speaking, when are learning differences identified?

Usually 3rd grade or later

A very bright kid with learning differences is often not identified until what grade?

7th –
The academic and organizational requirements usually increase significantly in 7th grade

Can social problems be classified as learning differences?

No (although they can impact social interactions)

Can evaluations of "failure to thrive" (FTT) be successfully conducted in the outpatient setting?

Usually not

Is FTT usually due to problems intrinsic to the child or due to environmental factors?

Environmental factors –
Nutrition, feeding techniques, appropriate social interactions, etc.

There are three ways a child can meet the criteria for FTT, based on a single piece of growth data information. What are those three criteria? (one criterion for weight percentile, two types of weight for height)

- Weight <3rd percentile
- Weight for height <5th percentile
- Weight ≥20 % below ideal for height

For very young infants, in the first 3 months of life, weight gain of less than how many grams = FTT?

<20 g per day

For infants between 3 and 6 months of age, weight gain of less than how many grams = FTT?

<15 g per day

We are used to thinking of FTT in terms of kids "falling off" their growth curve. How does that criterion work?

**Downward crossing of *two* major percentiles on the growth curve = FTT
Mnemonic:
FTT has two T's. The criterion is Falling Two percentiles**

Should environmental (nonorganic) causes of FTT be evaluated at the initial visit for FTT, or only after organic causes are ruled out?

Initial evaluation
(This is a change from past recommendations)

What is the most common general reason for FTT?

Inadequate amount of calories or inappropriate types of food intake

Which FTT patients definitely require inpatient evaluation? (4 groups)

- **Unstable or severely malnourished patients (of course!)**
- **Evidence of abuse of neglect**
- **High risk for abuse or neglect**
- **Outpatient management has failed**

Which FTT patients should be considered at "high risk" for abuse or neglect? (3 groups)

- **Very stressed home environment**
- **Parent–child interaction very abnormal**
- **Caregiver with very poor function**

Which pattern of childrearing puts the child at the highest risk for school phobia?

Single caretaker (including mom)

If a child has school phobia, what will usually work to calm the child?

Caretaker should accompany the child and gradually decrease the amount of time he/she stays (assuming that the phobia is related to separation)

What are the three main concerns regarding television viewing by children, according to the pediatric board exam?

1. Encourages inactivity
2. Increases children's difficulty separating fantasy & reality
3. Makes violence seem commonplace (more acceptable)

At what age is a child's sexual orientation able to be determined (at least for the board exam)?

Mid-adolescence

Is depression common in children?

Yes –
Especially likely if mood is interfering with daily functioning

When do night terrors occur, compared to when the child went to sleep?

Early –
First 1/3 of the night

When do night terrors occur, in terms of the sleep cycle?	They disrupt stage 4 non-REM sleep (kid looks awake, but fails to respond to outside stimulation)
Are there any clues in the family history to the probability that your patient has night terrors?	Yes – Family history is often positive for night terrors in other family members *(night terrors are more common in males)*
Are children with night terrors at risk to hurt themselves?	**Yes, because they are sometimes able to move during the episode**
How are night terrors treated?	Parental reassurance
Recurrent nightmares suggest stress in the child's life. Do night terrors also indicate stress?	No
Nightmares occur during which sleep stage?	**REM**
Are children with nightmares at risk for hurting themselves?	**Generally not**
If you wake an agitated child, how can you tell whether the child was having a nightmare or a night terror?	**Nightmares are remembered – Night terrors are not**
Which child is likely to be disoriented upon waking – the one having a nightmare, or the one having a night terror?	**Night terror**
Does talking during sleep indicate a sleep problem?	No
Does sleepwalking have a relationship to night terrors?	Yes – Both occur during stage 4 non-REM sleep
Is sleepwalking common in children?	Yes – 15 % will do it (most common between ages 4 and 8 years)

What physical findings do you expect for children having a night terror?	**Sympathetic nervous system stuff – Sweaty, dilated pupils, deep & rapid breathing, tachycardic**
What is the recommended way to handle a child having a night terror?	**Observe** (do not try to wake them)
What is the best management for sleepwalking?	**Lead the child back to bed & keep the environment safe**
What is the recommended way to handle nightmares?	Reassurance that the dream is over & the child is safe
What is "preemptive waking?"	Waking the child up just before the typical time for a night terror or sleepwalking episodes – Will sometimes prevent them
Do children with ADD or ADHD outgrow the disorder? *ADD = Attention-deficit disorder* *ADHD = Attention-deficit hyperactivity disorder*	About ½ will
Which gender develops ADD/ADHD more often?	**Boys**
Does limiting the sugar in the diet, or other dietary changes, improve the symptoms of ADD/ADHD?	**No**
What are the main symptoms of ADD/ADHD?	• Impulsiveness • Disorganization • Difficulty regulating attention (can be inattentive or overabsorbed, depending on the activity)
For someone who has never experienced ADD/ADHD, what is the best way to remember the symptom constellation?	They are much like sleep deprivation!
If a child behaves appropriately at the office visit, and seems bright, does this make ADD/ADHD less likely?	**No – Symptoms are less obvious in new or stimulating settings**

ADD/ADHD must be present by what age to make the diagnosis?	**Age 6 years – Although the diagnosis can be made retrospectively**
If an adolescent presents for the first time with acting out behavior and decreased attentiveness to school activities, is ADD/ADHD a likely diagnosis?	**No – Think substance abuse (or possibly anxiety/depression)**
Are salicylates a cause of attentional disorders?	No
Haven't some children with ADHD been shown to improve with a reduction in artificial colorings in their food?	NO!
Is the cause of ADD/ADHD known?	No
How is ADHD different from ADD?	Motor overactivity (fidgeting) is also present
A teacher sends a child for evaluation, because although he seems to be a bright student, he consistently fails to turn in his homework assignments, and often fails to follow instructions on the ones he does complete. Is this consistent with ADD?	Yes
Does emotional lability go along with attention deficit disorder?	It can – Same general idea as impulse control (emotions are not as well governed as usual, either)
Which treatments have proven efficacy for ADD/ADHD?	**Mainly stimulants & sometimes tricyclic antidepressants or clonidine (for hypervigilant & aggressive children)**
What is the main, general mechanism for ADD/ADHD medications?	Increased amounts of dopamine & norepinephrine

Why would stimulating
a hyper-stimulated kid be a helpful
therapy?

PET studies show that the prefrontal
area of the brain (planning,
sequencing, & impulse control)
is underactive in these patients –
With amphetamine-type medications, the prefrontal activity
increases

**Is there any down side to treating
ADD/ADHD kids with stimulants?**

**Yes –
Possible growth suppression
(anorexia, sleep difficulties) &
worsening of tic disorders
(if present)**

Which seizure disorder can sometimes
be confused for ADD?

Absence seizures

Are automatisms part of ADD/ADHD?

No –
That would be a seizure disorder

Which endocrine disorder should
be ruled out, if you are considering
an ADHD diagnosis?

Hyperthyroidism

Which environmental metals
can produce similar findings
to ADD/ADHD?

Lead (too much)
&
Iron (too little)

You would feel very foolish if you
diagnosed a child with ADD,
and then later discovered that he/she
actually had what problem?

Vision or hearing problems!!!
Always rule them out first

**If a child seems to have ADHD,
but the symptoms began at age
10 years, can you still make this
diagnosis?**

**No –
*Symptoms have to be present
by age 6 years!*

When children have a change
in behavior, and are less attentive
than usual, what iatrogenic cause must
always be considered?

Meds on board
(antihistamines, some antiseizure
meds, etc.)

How can you calculate the expected height for girls, based on the parents' heights?

Add mother's + father's height Subtract 13 cm (from the total) then divide by 2
(called the midparental height)

How is the calculation for a boy's expected height done, based on the parents' heights?

Add mother's + father's height ADD 13 cm (to the total) Then divide by 2

Developmentally speaking, how can you rule out colic as a cause of crying?

Age – If the child is >4 months, it is *not colic!*

What percentage of children should sleep through the night (about 5 h) by age 3 months?

About 50 %

Persistent disrupted sleep patterns in infants are linked to what frequent caregiver behaviors?

- Nighttime feeding after 6 months
- Caregiver responds to minor waking episodes during the night

When does the AAP recommend discontinuing overnight infant feedings (if the infant is not sleeping through the night)?

4–6 months

Does the AAP recommend having the infant sleep in the same room as the caregivers?

No

Should infants be put to bed after they have already fallen asleep, or allowed to fall asleep in their cribs on their own?

In their cribs (hopefully when they look sleepy, though!)

What is the most important factor in getting school-aged children to sleep successfully?

Bedtime routine

At what age should a child speak in complete sentences?

3 years

Should you worry about breath holding spells?

No – No long-term effects at all

What if a child turns pale and passes out during a breath holding spell? What should you worry about then?	Nothing, physically
What if a breath holding child turns blue, or passes out and has jerking movements like a seizure?	No risk of harm (unless they hit their head on the way to the ground!)
If a breath holding kid passes out, when in the course of the breath holding spell does that usually happen?	Breath holding is usually followed by a serious episode of crying – If syncope occurs, it is usually just after the crying begins
Can you inherit breath holding spells?	Oddly enough, yes – They seem to be autosomal dominant
During which ages are temper tantrums most common?	Ages 2–5 years
How common are daily tantrums for 2-year-olds?	20 %!!!
For the board exam, is any sort of physical punishing (for example, spanking) okay?	**No**
Which two developmental milestones are the hallmarks of development from 7- to 9-month-olds?	• **Sitting without support** • **Stranger anxiety begins**
At what age is separation anxiety most noticeable in infants & toddlers?	**9–18 months (can develop anytime after about 6 months)**
Separation anxiety should be largely gone by what age?	**Around 3 years**
The "avoidant" attachment pattern between a young child and his/her caregiver means that the child does what when the caregiver leaves and returns?	Leaves – Does not notice Returns – Moves away & continues to play

When children play in each other's company (besides each other), but do not actually interact, it is called "parallel play." Parallel play is most common between what ages?	1–3 years old
At what age do kids switch from parallel play to cooperative play?	**At approximately 3 years old**
What is the earliest age for normal toilet training?	18 months
What is the *usual* age range for toilet training?	**About 3 years old**
How old are kids when they develop "object permanence?" (Child knows that the object is still there, even if it is out of sight)	1–2 years old
How old are children when they can (usually) tell fantasy from reality?	Roughly 5 years
When do children usually develop a conscience?	Between 6 and 11 years
At what age is abstract reasoning possible?	Approximately 12 years (often develops later, though)
What is "truancy?"	**"Truancy" is the stereotype we think of with older kids "skipping school" –** **They are not at home (usually) or at school, and the caregivers do not know they are out of school**
How is "truancy" different from "school refusal?"	**In school refusal the child stays home, and the caregivers are aware**
What age group is most likely to "refuse school?"	Teenagers

Which gender most often refuses
to go to school?

Boys

**Children with school refusal issues
usually have what other sorts
of complaints?**

**Somatic –
Stomach aches, headaches,
anxiety, etc.**

If a child is upset and refuses
to go to school 1 day, is this a case
of "school refusal?"

No –
Must happen over 2 weeks, and
result in missing school 2–3 days
each week

What is the recommended management
for school refusal?

Set high expectations for the child
attending school, even if physical
complaints are present

**Do normal kids engage in head
banging?**

**Yes –
About 10 % of normal kids do**

**What about kids who sit and rock?
That often goes with neurological
impairment. Is it also seen
in normal kids?**

**Yes –
Up to 20 % do this at age 6
months**
(most stop by 3 years)

If a child starts to head bang or rock,
but appears to be otherwise normal,
is further evaluation for a neurological
problem indicated?

No

**What is the most common time
of the day for children to rock
(themselves) or head bang?**

Bedtime
(and sometimes in the middle of the
night)

**When can you expect thumb
sucking to stop?**

Usually by age 4 years
(But it can start in utero!)

**Which gender is more likely
to keep sucking on the thumb
into adolescence?**

Girls
(worrisome for underlying
psychological issues)

**Should children be discouraged
from sucking their thumbs?**

Not until they are 4 years old
(most stop spontaneously,
and there is no harm done)

Can thumb sucking cause any physical problems?

After 4 years old, it can lead to dental/palatal problems

Which method is most recommended for discouraging thumb sucking in an older child?

Positive reinforcement when the child is not thumb sucking

Do aversive techniques to discourage thumb sucking work?
(For example, putting nasty tasting stuff on the thumb)

Often, yes

What is onychophagia?

Nail biting

Which gender does more nail biting?

Boys, actually
(goes a little against the stereotype!)

How common is nail biting in adult men?

About 15 %

In school-aged children, before adolescence, which gender does more "onychophagia?"

Equal

What is bruxism, and why should a pediatrician be concerned about it?

- Grinding of teeth
- Can damage the teeth & bone over time, and also causes headache

Is masturbation in a young child unusual behavior?

**No –
It virtually always occurs**

If the topic comes up, what would the AAP like pediatricians to tell young children about masturbation?

That it is common & to keep it private

Is it common for young children to masturbate with objects other than their fingers or other very conveniently available objects?

No –
This should raise concern about sexual abuse

If parents object to masturbation, what would the AAP like the pediatrician to counsel them?

**Avoid punishments or other negative reactions –
Encourage redirecting behavior**

Does masturbation cause physical or mental problems?	No
In what age group is "exhibitionist" behavior of their nude bodies common?	3–6 years
Is it common for very young children (toddlers) to examine or touch each other's genitals?	Yes
Is it unusual for sexual play in children to include using the mouth to touch the genitals?	**Yes – may indicate abuse**
Is it common for young children to imitate sexual intercourse in their sexual play?	**Not in Western cultures** (in some cultures where children are more likely to see others engaging in intercourse, this would be more likely)
Do children typically act out sexual behaviors observed on television or from movies?	Generally, no
If a child's sexual play includes penetration, or discussion of intercourse, even with dolls, should you be worried about sexual abuse?	**Yes**
If a child is developmentally delayed, what should you expect with regard to their sexual play & exploration?	It will follow their developmental age (so it may be different from age-matched peers)
If a preschool child includes genitals on a drawing, should you be concerned about it?	No – That is common
If an elementary school-aged child includes genitals on a drawing, should you be concerned?	**Yes – It is not diagnostic of abuse, but is worth evaluating further** (depends on cultural background, also)

In cases of sexual abuse, is the abuser typically male or female?	**Male**
In cases of sexual abuse, is the abuser typically known to the victim, or a stranger?	**Known to the victim**
In cases of physical abuse, who is the most likely abuser?	**Female primary caregiver**
Is it normal for children & adolescents to be interested in pornography?	Yes, but the interest is usually limited
Is cross-dressing alright in preschool children?	Yes, it is common
At what age will children usually refuse to wear underwear of the "wrong" gender?	By age 5 years
What is "gender-identity disorder?"	**Believing you are of the opposite sex, trapped in the wrong body**
Do most homosexual people have gender-identity disorder?	**No –** **They are usually happy with their gender, but are also attracted to that same gender**
Are "tomboy" girls likely to have gender-identity disorder?	**No –** **Neither are more effeminate boys**
Do people with gender-identity disorder wish to literally change their gender to the opposite sex?	**Yes**
Is gender-identity disorder the same as transvestism (cross-dressing)?	No – In most cases, cross-dressing is done for sexual stimulation. Gender-identity disorder is about identity, not sexual excitement
Core gender identity is formed by what age?	3 years

We have all heard about children whose gender must be reassigned, after the child was initially thought to be the other gender. How long do you have to successfully reassign gender?

**Up to 3 years –
After gender identity is formed, it usually cannot be changed** (reassignment is, of course, not always successful before age 3)

Have the children of homosexual parents been found to have any negative effects due to being raised by homosexual parents?

No

Have children in two-caregiver households been found to have better development, on the average, than those in single-parent households?

Yes

How is being a gay or a lesbian adolescent linked to homelessness?

About 1/3 of homeless adolescents are homosexual

In terms of the available research, and the position of the AAP, does therapy to turn a gay or a lesbian adolescent into a heterosexual a good approach to try?

No, it is contraindicated (more likely to have psychological difficulties due to the lack of acceptance)

Roughly, what percentage of the population is homosexual?

Between 1 and 10 % (studies vary)

What is the most common recurring pain syndrome in children?

Headache

Which gender is more likely to complain of abdominal pain?

Girls

What proportion of children reports abdominal pain lasting 2 weeks or longer?

1/3!!!

If abdominal pain is "nonorganic" what important aspects of the exam will be normal?

Growth & development

Is it common for children with recurrent abdominal pain to have an organic cause?	**No – only about 5 % do**
How common is chest pain in children?	**Common – Especially in adolescents** *(Cardiac causes are very rare – most are psychogenic)*
What are "growing pains?"	Dull, aching pain in the limbs, usually the legs, with no obvious cause
Do growing pains require treatment?	No – They resolve with rest (usually overnight)
Are growing pains related to periods of rapid growth?	No *(cause is completely unknown)*
Which age group and gender most often has growing pains?	Around 10 years old & Female
What is the most common cause of musculoskeletal pain in children?	**Growing pains!**
If a new baby is expected in the household, what is the most helpful intervention for the older sibling?	**Increased attention to the older child from the father or other relative**
The upgoing Babinski reflex should disappear by what age?	**1 year**
Infants are born with a reflex that makes them grasp objects put into their palms. By what age should this reflex disappear?	**3 months** (known as palmar or palmar grasp reflex)

By what age should a child develop the "parachute" reflex?

6–9 months
Mnemonic:
You know this reflex must develop at about this time, because children need it *before* they start to walk – to protect themselves from fall injuries when they learn to walk!

What is the Moro reflex?

Sudden, upper extremity extension & abduction, then flexion with adduction, when the infant is falling backward

Should newborns have a Moro reflex?

Yes
(If it is absent, it is *very* worrisome)

By what age should the Moro reflex disappear?

By 5–6 months

Chapter 2
Neonatal Physiology: Things That Make Them Special!

Circulatory System

Neonates have a higher percentage of fluid in their body weight than older kids and adults. In addition to the general fluids guidelines for pediatrics there is a special adjustment for neonates.

Compute the maintenance fluids required, then decrease it by 1/3 on the first day of life, and by 1/4 on the second day. This is because neonates have a natural diuresis to reduce their fluid content toward normal in the first week of life. (You wouldn't want to overload them as they are trying to decrease their fluid content.)

Also, neonatal hearts are not able to increase stroke volume very well. If a neonate needs to increase oxygen delivery, it will increase the heart rate.

Fetal Circulation

Within the first 24 h, neonates are switching from fetal circulation to mature circulation. If the infant is overly stressed by something (such as sepsis, meconium aspiration, or pulmonary hypoplasia) they may fail to switch. This is called **P**ersistent **F**etal **C**irculation (**PFC**) and **P**ersistent **P**ulmonary **H**ypertension of the **N**ewborn (**PPHN**).

The circulatory differences:

In fetal life the lungs are not aerated, so blood supply to them is minimal (the pulmonary vascular resistance is high).

Because the pulmonary bed has high resistance, pressure in the right heart is actually higher than in the left heart. This pushes most of the blood through the foramen ovale. Blood which enters the pulmonary artery usually crosses over to the aorta through the patent ductus arteriosus for the same reason (high pulmonary vascular pressures).

C.M. Houser, *Pediatric Development and Neonatology: A Practically Painless Review*, 27
DOI 10.1007/978-1-4614-8681-7_2, © Springer Science+Business Media New York 2014

When the infant is born, the low-pressure placental system is suddenly removed from the circuit. The lung is aerated, which suddenly drops the pressure in the pulmonary bed.

The increased oxygen tension as the blood circulates by the PDA stimulates it to constrict and close within 24 h.

If fetal circulation persists, a vicious cycle is formed.

Treatment for this cycle is ventilation with a target of >90 % oxygen saturation & normal pH.

Systemic vasodilators are not very helpful because they are not specific to the pulmonary bed, but rather tend to dilate vessels everywhere. This is likely to produce overall hypotension—not good. An alternative pulmonary-vascular-specific therapy is inhaled pulmonary vasodilator nitric oxide, but this treatment is mainly useful for infants with reversible PPHN who also have normal left heart function. (A fixed PPHN lesion, such as in pulmonary hypoplasia or some congenital heart disorders, may not respond to inhaled nitric oxide.)

Respiratory System

New terminal bronchioles and alveoli are added until age 8 years. Lungs in even normal infants and young children have less capacity relative to overall size than adults.

Preemies have fewer Type #2 pneumocytes—these are the ones that make surfactant. Lack of surfactant leads to:

1. Alveolar collapse
2. Hyaline membrane formation
3. Decreased gas exchange

Renal System

Infants have a poor concentrating ability and a low GFR (glomerular filtration rate).

As mentioned above, term infants lose 5–10 % (and preterm 10–15 %) of their body weight in the first week of life due to natural diuresis.

Hepatic System

Drug metabolism is altered—the younger the child the more altered it is likely to be. This means that medications may accumulate much faster in a neonate or infant than you would expect.

Endocrine System

Most responses including the response to stressors are similar, but the success of the response may be limited because the energy stores (which the endocrine system is trying to mobilize) are so limited in young infants.

Temperature Regulation

Large BSA (body surface area) makes it hard to maintain the core body temperature.

Infants generate heat mainly from metabolism of brown fat rather than through shivering.

Chapter 3
Brief Overview of Reproductive Embryology

External genitalia – The external genitalia includes the penis or clitoris, the scrotal sac or labia majora/minora, and the lower 2/3 of the vagina. These structures begin as general structures that can differentiate into either male or female structures. If significant amounts of testosterone are not present, the differentiation will be female.

The clitoris or penis begins as the "genital tubercle." There are two ridges with folds on the perineum that develop into either the scrotal sac or labia. The lower portion of the vagina is formed by adjacent tissue from the urogenital sinus. The external genitalia differentiate into the male form due to local secretion of testosterone by the testes. This differentiation occurs around week 12 of gestation.

Internal reproductive structures – The internal structures of the male reproductive system develop from the mesonephric (aka wolffian) ducts. The internal structures of the female reproductive system (including the upper 1/3 of the vagina) are derived from the paramesonephric (aka mullerian) ducts. Male fetuses secrete mullerian inhibiting substance (MIS, sometimes written as mullerian inhibiting factor) which prevents development of the mullerian duct structures. If an otherwise normal male fetus lacks MIS, normal male development will continue, but the mullerian ducts will also mature into the female structures. Development of the wolffian structures is under genetic control.

Gonads – Stem cells for gonads begin on the wall of the yolk sac and progress to the abdominal cavity to complete their development. They later descend into the pelvis (ovaries) or scrotum (testes). The gubernaculum and processus vaginalis are connective tissues and a peritoneal evagination, respectively, that are important in the descent of the gonads. In the male these later become the gubernaculums testes and the tunica vaginalis. In the female they become the ovarian and round ligament of the uterus.

Pseudointersexuality – Medical designations of gender are based on the chromosomal gender, so female pseudointersexuality refers to individuals who are

C.M. Houser, *Pediatric Development and Neonatology: A Practically Painless Review*,
DOI 10.1007/978-1-4614-8681-7_3, © Springer Science+Business Media New York 2014

genetically XX, but who also have some male sexual characteristics. Male pseudointersexuality would refer to XY individuals with some female characteristics.

Female pseudointersexuality is the same as female hermaphroditism (only the name has changed) – These individuals are genetically XX, but some unusual source of androgens was present during fetal development such that the external genitalia develop partly or completely into male structures. (When androgens are present the external genitalia assume that this is due to the development of testicles and differentiate into male structures.) The internal structures will be normal female reproductive structures.

The usual cause of this problem is either exogenous androgens (in medications, for example) or adrenal hyperplasia of the fetus itself, in which the adrenal secretes unusual quantities of testosterone.

Male pseudointersexuality (same as male hermaphroditism) – As mentioned above, if a genetically male fetus does not secrete adequate quantities of mullerian inhibiting substance, female internal reproductive structures will develop along with the male structures. If the fetus fails to produce adequate quantities of testosterone, the external genitalia will fail to fully differentiate into the male structures.

Testicular feminization syndrome (aka androgen insensitivity syndrome) – This syndrome occurs when a genetically male fetus lacks androgen receptors. Although the testes secrete hormone appropriately, the external genitalia takes no notice. Although these individuals function as females in society, they lack female internal reproductive structures as the mullerian-inhibiting substance is still secreted normally (preventing development). The undescended testes are usually removed to prevent the development of testicular cancer, which frequently develops in undescended testes.

Chapter 4
Cryptorchidism and Contraindications to Breast Feeding in Developed Nations

Cryptorchidism

- Should be placed into the scrotum by about 12 months.
- Moving them to the scrotum does not change the cancer risk (although it does alter the type of cancer that is likely to develop). (*Please note that information on this topic is frequently incorrect. The above point has been checked* and *double-checked. It is correct to the best of current knowledge.*)
- Moving them to the scrotum dramatically improves later fertility.
- Some testes come down on their own, usually in the first 3–6 months. For babies born with undescended testes, 90 % of preterm and 75 % of full-term will descend on their own by 9 months.
- There are some hormonal treatments that can be tried for *bilateral* cryptorchidism, but they are not very successful.

Contraindications to Breast Feeding in Developed Nations

- Active TB (possible aerosol spread)
- Breast cancer treatments – radioactive agents, cyclosporine, methotrexate, some other specific chemotherapy agents
- Street drug use (cocaine, PCP)
- Lithium
- HTLV 1 or 2
- HIV
- HSV lesions on breast
- Galactosemia

C.M. Houser, *Pediatric Development and Neonatology: A Practically Painless Review*,
DOI 10.1007/978-1-4614-8681-7_4, © Springer Science+Business Media New York 2014

Chapter 5
Neonatal Topics

What is the most common complication of NG feeding in infants?

Diarrhea

What is the second most common complication of NG feeding in infants?

Reflux

What general type of formula is best for NG feeding?

Elemental
(reduces complications)

What is the <u>worst</u> complication of NG feeding (at any age)?

Aspiration

When should *bolus* NG feeding be used?
(assuming it is well tolerated)

In cases of oral-motor dyscoordination

Why is continuous NG feeding preferred for Crohn's patients?
(2 reasons)

Increases probability of remission
&
May overcome growth failure

What type of NG feeding is preferred for infants with congenital heart disease (and why)?

Continuous –
High nutritional demand & delayed gastric emptying

If an infant has a malabsorption syndrome, what type of NG feeding schedule is best?

Continuous

C.M. Houser, *Pediatric Development and Neonatology: A Practically Painless Review*,
DOI 10.1007/978-1-4614-8681-7_5, © Springer Science+Business Media New York 2014

For the boards, breast feeding is generally superior to any other infant food. What deficiencies, though, does breast milk have?	**Low vitamin K** **Low protein** **Low iron** **Low calcium** *(But absorption of iron is better from breast milk than from other sources)*
Healthy newborns should "deliver" their first stool in what amount of time?	**48 h** **(99 % within 24 h)**
If a child does not have a stool in the first 48 h after birth, what two diagnoses should you rule-out first?	**1. Hirschsprung's** **2. Cystic fibrosis**
Polyhydramnios is linked to what pancreatic cause of vomiting in the newborn?	**Annual pancreas**
Progressive (worsening), non-bilious vomiting in the first month of life – especially in a male – suggests what structural problem?	**Pyloric stenosis**
A neonate with *vomiting, lethargy, low sodium, and low pH*, may have what important endocrine disorder? *(highly tested item)*	**Adrenal insufficiency**
Polyhydramnios with copious oral secretions after birth, along with inability to pass a feeding tube, suggests what diagnosis?	**Tracheo-esophageal fistula**
What type of tracheo-esophageal fistula is most common?	**Blind esophageal pouch with distal esophageal fistula Type C**
How do patients with tracheo-esophageal fistulas appear at first feeding?	They usually cough & may become cyanotic
How commonly does meconium (ileus) plug syndrome occur in CF patients?	Only 10 %
Aside from obstruction, what is the other bad complication of meconium plug syndrome?	Perforation

What neurologically-based disorders make meconium plugs in the newborn more likely?	**Hirschsprung's (rectal aganglionosis)**
What medication or drug-related situations make meconium plugs more likely? (2)	• **Illicit maternal drug use (especially opiates)** • **Maternal magnesium sulfate treatment**
What endocrine-related disorders make meconium plugs more likely?	• **Hypothyroidism** • **Small left-colon syndrome (associated with maternal diabetes)**
What causes meconium plugs, anyway?	Less water than usual in the meconium
What is meconium plug *syndrome?*	Functional immaturity of the colon's ganglion cells causes failure to pass meconium
How is meconium plug syndrome treated?	Enema evacuation of the meconium is usually sufficient
Is meconium plug *syndrome* associated with cystic fibrosis?	No!
What is meconium ileus, as opposed to a meconium plug?	**Meconium ileus is lower intestinal obstruction due to meconium – There may or may not be an especially dense "plug"**
On the boards, meconium ileus = what disorder, most of the time? *(popular test item!)*	**CF**
Why do CF kids have a higher risk for meconium ileus?	Their meconium is more viscous, due to a higher albumin content
Where does the obstruction usually occur in meconium ileus?	**The *terminal ileum***
The abdominal exam of an infant with meconium ileus can often be described with what "buzzword?"	**"Doughy" (because the gut is full of meconium instead of air & fluid)**

How is meconium ileus treated?

Enemas are used to draw water into the gut (refluxing into the terminal ileum)
(Gastrografin/Hypaque or hypertonic barium enemas may be used)

What must you be very careful of when treating meconium ileus with an enema?

Fluid shifts → shock

Which infants will need surgical management of their meconium ileus? (3 situations)

"Complicated" meconium ileus:
• Perforation
• Volvulus, or
• Atresia

What is the appearance of meconium on X-ray?

"Ground glass" or "bubbly"

What is the first thing you should think of in a newborn with lower GI blood?

Whether the blood could be ingested maternal blood

What test is used to differentiate the origin of lower GI blood (maternal or infant)?

The "apt" test

What disorders of the neonate/newborn are likely to cause lower GI bleeding? (3)

1. Necrotizing enterocolitis (especially preemies)
2. Hirschsprung's (with associated colitis)
3. Malrotation with volvulus (also presents with vomiting)

What is the most common cause of cholestatic jaundice for neonates?

TPN
(total parenteral nutrition)
Especially common in the premature

If a newborn has contracted neonatal hepatitis, when will that disease present?

**Months later
(Usually 2–6 months later, except hepatitis A which presents sooner)**

**What causes elevated direct bilirubin in neonates?
(two options)**

**Either
Anatomical/obstructive problems
  Or
Parenchymal liver disease**

What is cholestatic jaundice?

Elevated direct bilirubin due to inability to get the bile *out*

In a jaundiced child, what lab values can help can you distinguish cholestatic from hepatocellular causes?

Cholestatic – high alk phos
Cellular – high AST & ALT

When does biliary atresia usually present (jaundice, high direct bili)?

After age 1 month

How can you easily calculate the caloric requirements of a healthy infant?

100 kcal × first 10 kg +
50 kcal × second 10 kg +
20 kcal/kg for all remaining kg

Can premature infants get all of their nutrition from breast milk?

No –
Protein supplements are needed

How is the breast milk produced in the beginning of a feeding different from the milk produced at the end?

"Hind" milk (produced at end) is higher in *fat & protein, & lower in lactose*

How is colostrum different from regular breast milk?

High in:
Protein
Carotene (yellow color)
GI-related enzymes

Why are premature infants at risk for fat-soluble vitamin deficiencies?

They have less bile acid production, so fat absorption is difficult

Is the breast milk produced by a preterm mother significantly different compared to that of a full-term mother?

Less milk is usually produced, but it has more protein & electrolytes.

(Inadequate protein, calcium, phosphorous, and Vitamin D means that supplementing breast milk with human milk fortifier is needed to provide adequate growth and nutrition for preterm infants)

How much protein do premature infants require per day?

3.5 g/kg

How much protein do full-term infants require per day?

About 2 g/kg

How much weight gain should a full-term infant average (after the initial drop in weight)?	20–30 g/day
How quickly should a preemie be expected to gain weight?	15–20 g/day
How do we define LGA (large for gestational age), both by weight and by growth chart percentile for term infants?	• >3,900 g • Upper 10th percentile
How do we define SGA (small for gestational age), both by weight and by growth chart percentile for term infants?	• <2,500 g • Lowest 10th percentile
When does "periodic breathing" become apnea?	When it lasts more than 15 s (20 s, according to some sources)
How is a full-term birth defined?	Delivery between 38 and 42 weeks
If a child has a low initial Apgar score, but a normal 5-min Apgar, what is the child's prognosis?	**Normal**
At 5 min after birth, what two factors increase the risk of infant mortality for *preterm* infants?	Persistent bradycardia & Apgar <4
Should you use the 1-min Apgar score to decide whether to initiate CPR?	**No –** **If the child meets CPR criteria, start immediately!**
Bilateral ankle clonus in a newborn infant suggests what problem?	None – It can be a normal finding at that age
What is a normal scalp pH?	**7.25** **(<7.2 is worrisome)**
Home-birthed infants are at special risk for what two problems?	**Sepsis** **&** **Vitamin K deficiency** **(producing bleeding/hemorrhage)**
Does acrocyanosis require intervention in the newborn?	No

The two most common causes of fetal demise are…?	**Chromosomal abnormality** & **Congenital malformations**
What is the best initial test to evaluate an anuric newborn?	Renal ultrasound
Is it preferable to place erythromycin ointment or silver nitrate drops into the newborn's eyes?	**Erythromycin** (It is less irritating – although it is a little less certain to kill all bacteria. For Chlamydia, long-term treatment is needed)
What is the most common reason for a seizure occurring in the first 24 h after birth?	**Birth hypoxia**
If a full-term neonate has a seizure due to birth hypoxia, what is his/her long-term neurological prognosis?	<u>**Normal**</u>
A bad episode of birth hypoxia can lead to what dreaded complication?	**Multisystem organ failure (MSOF!!!)**
Premature and "very low birth weight" infants often score no higher than 6 on the Apgar. Why?	**Minimal tone & minimal reflex irritability lower their scores –** *This is just due to an immature neurological system*
Very low birth weight neonates are at risk for hypothermia & hypoglycemia. Why?	Small muscle mass & fat stores mean little glycogen & brown fat is available
What does the fetal "non-stress test" measure?	**Appropriate change in fetal heart rate with fetal activity**
What test detects the amount of mixing (exposure) between fetal & maternal blood? (in the maternal circulation)	Kleihauer-Betke
What is normal hemoglobin for a full-term newborn?	≥ 13
What percentage of hemoglobin is fetal hemoglobin at the time of a full-term birth?	80 %

What is the typical pattern for the hemoglobin level in preterm infants?

Starts high ($\geq$13)
Then drops to nadir generally by 2 months before stabilizing
(The low value should be about 8 for preterm infants)

What is the typical pattern for the hemoglobin level in term infants?

Starts high
Then drops for 2–3 months before stabilizing
(The low value should be about 10)

How is the typical pattern for hemoglobin level different in preterm infants?
(3)

- **Their starting Hgb levels are lower**
- **Their low value is lower (7 or 8)**
- **They hit bottom sooner (1–2 months)**

What problems often accompany polycythemia?
(4)

1. Hypoglycemia (RBCs eat it up!)
2. Hyperbilirubinemia (too many RBCs break & spill Hgb)
3. Thrombocytopenia
4. Hyperviscosity syndrome

How should you test for polycythemia, if you suspect it?

<u>Central</u> venous blood is needed
(Other sources might be hemoconcentrated)

If a newborn is given vitamin K orally, will this provide equal protection against hemorrhage, compared to the IM injection?

No

What is "early onset" neonatal hemorrhage, now also known as early onset vitamin K deficiency bleeding?

Within the first 24 h of life
(typically described as bleeding from the cord or circumcision site)

Early onset vitamin K deficiency neonatal bleeding usually develops in infants whose mothers have used which types of medications?

Anticonvulsants & anti-tuberculosis medications

When does classic neonatal hemorrhage happen?

2–7 days after birth
(Usually infant has not received vitamin K supplementation)

What is "late onset" neonatal hemorrhage?

>1 week, but <6 months old
*(typically a breast-fed infant with diarrhea, whose K has gone low – **intrancranial bleeding most common in this group!**)*

If a birth mother has ITP, what can you expect to see in the newborn?
(ITP = idiopathic thrombocytopenia purpura)

**Thrombocytopenia –
It will *spontaneously improve*
in about 1 month**
(Mom's IgG against platelets crosses the placenta)

When does the umbilical cord stump normally fall off?

By 2 weeks of age

If the umbilical cord stump does not fall off by 1 month, what does this suggest?

**A neutrophil disorder
(could be a low count or defect in activity – neutrophils are in charge of getting rid of the stump!)**

Why should the baby be held below the cord for at least 30 s before clamping?

To prevent a decreased hematocrit (from cells being trapped in the cord)

The umbilical cord ordinarily has two arteries and one vein. If there is only *one* artery, what organ may also be abnormal?

**One or both kidneys
(Get an ultrasound to screen for kidney problems)**

What infectious complication do you worry about with umbilical vein catheterization?

Omphalitis
(belly button infection!)

Which vascular complications should you worry about, when catheterizing the umbilical vein or artery?
(4)

- Thrombosis
- Embolus
- Perforation/hemorrhage
- Compromise of the femoral artery (in the case of artery catheterization)

Is the liver at any risk with umbilical catheterization?

Yes –
Can cause necrosis or hemorrhage

What is "low" position for an umbilical artery catheter?

L3-5

What is "high" position for an umbilical artery catheter?	T 6-10
What are the two types of brachial plexus injury?	Erb's palsy & Klumpke's palsy
How can you recognize an infant with an Erb's palsy?	**The affected arm is positioned "like a waiter ready to receive a tip"** (assuming the waiter is being very discrete about picking up the tip – the arm is adducted, internally rotated, with wrist and fingers flexed toward the back)
Which brachial plexus nerve roots are damaged, in kids with Erb's palsy?	C5-7
Klumpke palsy causes what sort of hand appearance?	Claw hand Mnemonic: The hand looks like it's grabbing a "clump" of something
Which nerves are affected in Klumpke palsy?	C8-T1
What other anatomically related neurological disorder is sometimes seen with Klumpke palsy?	Horner's syndrome
What is the main way to distinguish an omophalocele from gastroschisis?	**An omphalocele is covered in a membrane** **(& sits in the middle of the belly)**
Omphalocele is especially associated with what congenital syndrome?	Beckwith-Wiedemann syndrome (Macroglossia, Macrosomia, Hypoglycemia)
What organs are involved in an omphalocele?	**Bowel & sometimes other organs (e.g., liver)**
On which side of the body do you see gastroschisis?	**The right**

**What organs are involved
in gastroschisis?**

**Generally just bowel
(& no membrane covering)**

**Which disorder is commonly associated
with chromosomal disorders –
omphalocele or gastroschisis?**

Omphalocele

How can you remember that omphaloceles
are the covered abdominal defect?

Imagine a big "O"-shaped cover
over the organs (They are membrane
covered)

How can you remember that omphaloceles
are associated with chromosomal
abnormalities?

Picture the gut loops inside
the "O" cover looking like little
chromosomes

High AFP level (alpha fetoprotein) is used
to screen for what antenatal abnormalities?

- Anencephaly & neural tube
  defects
- Abdominal wall defects &
  bladder extrophy
- Renal abnormalities

**Low AFP level is associated with
what common chromosomal disorder?**

Trisomy 21

**AFP can be falsely high if what
important piece of information
is incorrect?**

Gestational age

**What is included in the (antenatal)
"biophysical profile?"
(5 components)**

1. **Fetal movement**
2. **Reactive heart rate**
3. **Breathing**
4. **Tone**
5. **Amniotic fluid volume**

What is the significance of a birth-related
clavicle fracture?

None really –
it usually resolves on its own, and is
more common in larger babies

How is midgut volvulus diagnosed?

Upper GI series

Aside from vomiting/obstruction, what is
the danger of midgut volvulus?

Ischemia/necrosis of significant
amounts of bowel

How do you diagnose Hirschsprung's disease?	Biopsy (usually a suction biopsy from the rectum)
Aside from obstruction, what is the danger of Hirschsprung's disease?	Megacolon/perforation (of the segment just before the aganglionic area)
If an infant has a "scaphoid abdomen" and decreased breath sounds on the left, what is the diagnosis?	**Congenital diaphragmatic hernia (most are on the left side)**
Irritability, tremor, and SVT in the first 24-h after birth suggest what diagnosis?	Neonatal thyrotoxicosis
What causes neonatal thyrotoxicosis?	**Maternal antibodies that stimulate the thyroid**
How is neonatal thyrotoxicosis different from the presentation of inborn errors of metabolism or hormonal pathways?	**Inborn errors typically present later**
How high can a normal bilirubin be in a full-term newborn?	12.4
For breast-fed infants, bili levels usually peak at how many days of life?	**Four – & often stay up until day 6 or 7**
Which infants, especially on the boards, are most likely to develop objectionable levels of bilirubin? *(popular test item)*	**Breast-fed males <38 weeks gestation <72 h old (Remember that these babies have often been discharged to home before the bili peaks)**
If you are sending a newborn home, and the bilirubin has not yet reached its peak, what should you do?	**Screen the bilirubin** (get either a total or transcutaneous measurement), **Then, Plot it on a nomogram for hours of life to get the percentile**
The common pathological causes of high bilirubin in neonates are usually due to what general process?	Too much bili production of some sort (such as RBC destruction)

What medication can be used to stimulate bile secretion and decrease serum bilirubin?

Phenobarbital

When giving phototherapy, what color of light is most effective?

Blue – But it is seldom used due to eyestrain & other complications

Which light color is effective for bilirubin phototherapy, and has the best skin penetration?

Green

What color of light is most often used for bilirubin phototherapy?

Fluorescent white light

What is the goal in phototherapy for hyperbilirubinemia?

Reduce the level by about 5 (stop at that point)

When might an exchange transfusion be needed for a high bilirubin level?

If the bili is ≥30 & There are signs of ongoing hemolysis (or other reason for increase)

What are the four main complications should you worry about with exchange transfusion?

1. Low calcium
2. High potassium
3. Hypovolemia
4. Thrombocytopenia

Physiological jaundice of the newborn occurs during what period following birth?

Days 1–5 (not the first 24 h)

What does the term "breast-fed jaundice" refer to?

Jaundice in the *first week* of life – due to dehydration/low calorie intake

How is breast *milk* jaundice different from breast-*fed* jaundice?

Breast milk jaundice occurs >1 week after birth (occurs for complex reasons, but not due to dehydration) Mnemonic: "F" for "fed" comes before "M" for milk

What component of hyperalimentation causes cholestatic jaundice (mainly)?

The protein (limit to no more than 2 g/kg/day)

Will anything (other than Phenobarbital) increase bilirubin excretion in newborns?

Yes –
Increased frequency of feedings

Why does an increased number of oral feedings help the infant lower its bilirubin?

Increased excretion & reduced enterohepatic recirculation

If neonatal jaundice first occurs after the baby has already reached 1 week of age, what should you consider?
(4)

1. Sepsis (always)
2. Breast milk jaundice
3. Hypothyroid
4. Galactosemia
   (of course, there are other possibilities, but they are less likely or worrisome)

Persistent jaundice suggests what causes of neonatal jaundice?
(1 inborn error)
(1 anomaly)
(2 infectious)
(1 iatrogenic)

1. Galactosemia
2. TORCH diseases
3. Congenital atresia of the bile ducts
4. Hepatitis
5. Hyperalimentation or drug-related

Jaundice that develops between days 4 & 7 of life suggests what possible causes?

Infectious!!!
    In particular –
    1. Sepsis
    2. UTI
    3. TORCH infections or the noninfectious cephalohematoma

(Physiological jaundice also peaks during this time period, but it typically begins earlier)

At what bilirubin level should you begin phototherapy, if there is no evidence of hemolysis, & the baby is otherwise healthy?

15–20 mg/dL, depending on age
(15 up to 48 h old)
(18 up to 72 h old)
(20 if ≥72 h old)

Why is high bilirubin a problem?

Risk of CNS damage
(called "kernicterus")

Kernicterus is most likely to develop when an infant's high bilirubin level developed from what process?

Hemolysis

In "acute kernicterus," how many symptom phases do you see?

Three

Phase I kernicterus has what type of symptoms?

Low stuff, mainly –
- **Low tone (hypotonia)**
- **Low suck**
- **Low level of consciousness (stupor)**
+ Seizures (low neural inhibition)

The middle phase of acute kernicterus features what symptoms?

Overactivity/high stuff –
- **Hypertonia (in extensors)**
- **Opisthotonous (rigid back arching)**
- **Retrocollis**
+ Fever (overactive brain stem)

The final phase of acute kernicterus is simply hypertonia. What happens in the chronic phase?

It's a mix of high & low stuff –
Low stuff:
Hypotonia & delayed motor skills
High stuff:
Hyperactive deep tendon reflexes & tonic neck reflexes

If an infant with a history of high bili's is now hypertonic, but doesn't have fever or any funny posturing, what does the infant have?

Phase 3 (acute) kernicterus

Just to be sure you've remembered, at what bili level would you consider doing an exchange transfusion to lower the bilirubin?

$\geq$30 with signs of ongoing hemolysis (or some other reason for continuing increase)

In exchange transfusion, how much new blood is infused?
Note: This is not the same as a partial exchange transfusion, which can be done for polycythemia

Twice the circulating blood volume
(Because it is done a little at a time – so twice is given to ensure most of the old blood is gone)

**What CBC problem is common
in exchange transfusion?**

Low platelets

What is a Grade 1 hemorrhage?

Germinal matrix only

What is a Grade 2 hemorrhage, then?

Intraventricular hemorrhage *but
no dilation*

**What is a Grade 3 intracranial
hemorrhage?**

Intraventricular hemorrhage *with
dilation (of the ventricles)*

**What is a Grade 4 intracranial
hemorrhage?**

1. **Intraventricular hemorrhage**
2. **+Dilation**
3. **Parenchymal involvement**

**Why are the fluid requirements
of preterm infants higher than those
of full-term infants?**

Immature skin
   &
**Higher ratio of surface area
to body mass**
(More insensible fluid loss)

In a preterm infant, what are the upper
and lower limits of serum glucose?

150 & 40

**Is the glucose requirement of a preterm
infant greater or less than that of a
full-term infant?**

**Greater!
(6–8 mg/kg/min vs. 4–6
for full-term infants)**

When is it safe to add potassium to the IV
fluids of a neonate?
(2 criteria)

Urine output is adequate
   &
Potassium level <4.5

Should sodium be added to a newborn's
IV fluids?

Generally not needed until >72 h old

Is a preterm infant's sodium requirement
greater than or less than that of a full-term
infant?

Greater
(about 5 mEq/kg/day vs. 3)

Will most babies of ABO incompatible
mothers develop significant hemolysis?

No

If a neonate is hypoglycemic, is it alright
to bolus him or her?

Yes –
It's important!
(2 cc/kg of D_{10})

Why is IM glucagon usually not a good way to treat hypoglycemia in neonates and preemies?

Low muscle mass (no glycogen stores to release)

If a newborn is hypoglycemic after the mother has received tocolytics, how are the two related?

Tocolytics stimulate fetal insulin secretion!

In a hypocalcemic infant/neonate who is not responding to calcium repletion, what other level should be checked?

Magnesium (Normal Mg is needed for calcium repletion to work – same for potassium repletion)

Elevated neonatal levels of magnesium (due to Mg given to the mother) can cause a problem for another electrolyte. Which one?

Calcium (High magnesium suppresses PTH)

What are the two main clinical tests for low calcium levels?

Trousseau's (carpopedal spasm if you inflate the BP cuff) & Chvostek's (Tapping on the facial nerve produces a twitch) Mnemonic: Trousseau's sounds like "tourniquet," which reminds you of the BP cuff

What is the best lab test to evaluate possible hypocalcemia?

Ionized calcium (sent on ice)

A neonate with both pneumatosis intestinalis & air in the biliary tree is likely to have what diagnosis?

NEC (necrotizing enterocolitis)

Which portions of the gut are most commonly affected by NEC?

Distal ileum & Proximal colon

NEC usually presents during what period of life?

First 2 weeks

Which infants are at risk of NEC longer than the initial 2 weeks of life, sometimes developing NEC as late as 3 months old?

Babies born at <1,000 g

Is NEC infectious?

Not clear –
But most cases don't seem to be infectious

A baby who has had an episode of NEC should remain NPO for how long after the event?

Most stop feedings until at least 1 week after X-rays normalize
(evidence is unclear, at this time)

Aside from stopping all oral feeding, how else should you manage NEC, initially?
(3 steps)

1. NG decompression
2. Give IV fluid (of course), & fix any electrolyte issues
3. Get cultures, then start antibiotics (e.g., ampicillin & gentamicin)

Does feeding by catheter cause NEC?

No –
Never been proven in studies
(but it is still usually removed, as it could worsen the situation)

If a peritoneal tap shows pus or feces in a NEC infant, what is the recommended management?

Surgery

Medical management works in what proportion of NEC cases?

¾
(usually takes 2 weeks to resolve)

If you are considering treating a neonate with naloxone (Narcan®), what important historical data would you like to know about the mother?

Whether the mother is a chronic opiate user – if so, naloxone could cause seizures

Over what amount of time should a preemie's growth "catch up" with that of same aged peers?

The first 2 years

Some premature infants are at risk for retinopathy of prematurity (ROP) only if exposed to high oxygen levels. What defines this group?

30–35 weeks gestation
    &
Birth weight between 1,300 and 1,800 g

Which neonates are <u>always</u> at risk
to develop ROP?

<30 weeks gestation
  Or
<1,300 g
*(even without supplemental oxygen
exposure)*

When should infants be evaluated
for ROP?

At discharge, or at 4 weeks old
– whichever comes first

Why are preemies at risk to develop
rickets?

Their calcium/phosphorous intake is
often not adequate

Why do preemies need unusually large
amount of calcium & phosphorous?

Their gut absorbs very little
of either one
(risk of osteopenia/rickets)

Why do preemie formulas contain
medium chain triglycerides (MCTs)?

They are absorbed without
assistance from bile
(preemies have less bile)

How many calories per ounce are found
in preemie formula?

24 kcal/oz

Why do preemie formulas include
glucose polymers rather than lactose?

Better absorption
(and fewer reactions)

What is the optimal ratio of whey:
casein for preemie formula?

60:40
whey:casein

**If meconium is the cause of respiratory
distress, how will the infant present?**

Tachypnea
Intercostal retractions
+/– Cyanosis

**What is the most likely complication
of meconium aspiration syndrome,
long-term?**

**Persistent pulmonary
hypertension**

**What is the most important preventa-
tive measure in meconium births?**

**Suctioning before the infant's
body is delivered**

In a meconium delivery, is it necessary to
intubate when the meconium is thin, and
the baby seems well?

No –
No intervention needed
*(No visualization recommended
anymore)*

In a meconium delivery with thick meconium, and/or a "floppy" baby, what should you do?
(3 steps)

1. Suction the upper airway (only if needed to visualize, otherwise intubate patient with minimal stimulation)
2. Intubate
3. Suction the lower airway

For meconium babies, are prophylactic antibiotics helpful to decrease infection?

No
(although they are still often given)

How common are pneumothoraces/ pneumomediastinum in mechanically ventilated infants, especially those with meconium aspiration?

Common – About 15 % of ventilated patients

If pneumothoraces are small, and the infant is not in any distress, what should you do about it (whether the child had meconium or not)?

Nothing – Just watch the pneumothorax to be sure it decreases

Initial management of a symptomatic neonate with a pneumothorax is _____?

22-gauge angiocath in the 2nd intercostal space, mid-clavicular line (Decompresses it, if it is actually a tension pneumothorax)

Will most cases of pneumomediastinum require management?

No

If breast milk is frozen, then thawed, how quickly must it be used?

Within 48 h

Can a mother taking chemo or radiation treatment breast feed?

Generally, no

Should mothers with HSV (herpes simplex virus) lesions breast feed?

It's fine, as long as they don't have lesions on the breast

Should HIV infected mothers breast feed?

No

This disease, common among immigrants, is a contraindication to breast feeding. What is it?

TB (active forms – risk of transmission to the infant)

Is it alright for individuals with CMV infections to breast feed?

No

Are mothers with inborn errors of metabolism good candidates for breast feeding?

Generally not
(examples are PKU and galactosemia)

There are a variety of medications that are incompatible with breast feeding. What common endocrine condition's treatment falls into this group?

Hyperthyroid medications

A neonate with alopecia, thrombocytopenia, and scaly dermatitis may have what nutritional problem?

Essential fatty acid deficiency
(especially linoleic acid)

How is fatty acid deficiency treated?

IV lipids –
Especially linoleic acid

If a neonate presents with hemolytic anemia, thrombo-cytosis, and edema, what nutritional deficit should you suspect?

Vitamin E
Mnemonic:
E is for Edema
E is for Elevated platelets
E is for Erythrocyte problem
(Hemolytic anemia in a newborn should always make you consider vitamin E deficiency)

Dry skin, poor wound healing, and perioral rashes in a neonate suggest what nutritional deficiency?

Zinc
(Rash can also be perianal)

What ratio is used to determine risk for respiratory distress syndrome at birth?

The L:S ratio
(lecithin:sphingomyelin)

What is a good L:S ratio?

>2.0

The L:S ratio is used to predict fetal lung maturity, based on amniotic fluid findings. What single factor in amniotic fluid is a good predictor?

Phosphatidylglycerol

What common maternal condition often alters the L:S ratio?

Diabetes

What is surfactant made of?

Lecithin (65 %)
Cholesterol
Phosphatidylglycerol
Apoproteins (Surfactant proteins
SP-A, B, C, D)

Which cells make surfactant?

Type II pneumocytes
(aka alveolar cells)

What pH value suggests that the infant requires ventilation?

7.2

At what CO_2 value (from the ABG) would you consider ventilating a neonate?

>60

If a neonate is requiring 50 % FiO_2 to maintain a PaO_2 >50, what intervention should you consider?

Surfactant

Which infants are at highest risk
for hyaline membrane disease?
(gestational age, race, & gender)

Preterm
Caucasian
Males

A severely hypoxic neonate who does
not respond to O_2 has what kind
of problem (usually)?
(popular test item!)

Right to Left cardiac shunt
(including shunts through
the ductus)

Infants weighing <1,500 g are at special
risk for what problem if their pulmo-
nary resistance drops rapidly?

Shunting through a patent ductus
into **the lungs → pulmonary edema**

How is patent ductus arteriosus (PDA)
shunting that produces pulmonary
edema treated?

Ligation of the PDA
  Or
NSAIDs to chemically close it

Is the WBC count a reliable indicator of sepsis in a newborn?

No
(The normal range is very broad, and WBC response is unpredictable)

If a neonate is floppy & lethargic, what three general diagnoses should be considered first?

1. Sepsis
2. Congenital adrenal hyperplasia
3. Inborn errors of metabolism

Does congenital toxoplasmosis manifest itself in the neonatal period?

Generally not

Neonatal sepsis is most commonly caused by what organisms?

Group B Strep
&
E. Coli
(Listeria is less common, but must still be covered with antibiotics)

What CBC & coagulation parameters are often abnormal in infants with Group B Strep, early in the infection?
(3)

- Leucopenia
- Thrombocytopenia
- PT/PTT

Which sort of staph bacteria should be considered as a possible cause of neonatal sepsis?

Coagulase negative
(meaning staph *other than Staph aureus*)

A Group B strep infection that presents in the first few days of life typically causes which two types of infections (in addition to overall sepsis)?

Pneumonia
  Or
Meningitis

Group B strep infections that occur after the first few days of life most commonly cause which two specific types of infection, in addition to overall sepsis?

Osteomyelitis
  Or
Meningitis

On the boards, if you are shown a chest X-ray, and asked for the birth diagnosis, what common problem should you look for?
(frequently tested item!)

Fractured clavicle

In a twin birth, which twin is more likely to develop respiratory problems – the first or second born?

Second born

Are monozygotic or dizygotic twins more at risk for complications, in general?

Monozygotic
(Remember that monozygotics share both chorion & amnion)

Neonates with respiratory distress syndrome often require prolonged ventilation. This puts them at risk for what long-term complication?

Bronchopulmonary dysplasia

In general, how is bronchopulmonary dysplasia treated?

Fluid restriction
Diuretics
Bronchodilators

What electrolyte abnormality are BPD infants especially at risk for?

Hypocalcemia
(related to diuretic use)

Should you rely on the results of a dextrostrip test for glucose to guide your treatment?

**Generally no –
Combine with clinical impression until you can get a lab glucose**

Name two common causes of erroneous glucose results?

1. Sample drawn too close to IV site (can cause either low or high value)
2. Sample not on strip long enough (low value)

Folic acid supplementation is thought to decrease the incidence of neural tube defects by about what percentage?

50 %!

When is O_2 & stimulation likely to be sufficient to resuscitate a newborn?

With first time (primary) apnea

If primary apnea is not treated, what is the natural course of this problem?

Another round of gasping will begin, followed by another (secondary) apnea

How is secondary apnea of the newborn treated?

Ventilation only

What is the first thing to think of, when a ventilated patient begins to desaturate (lose O_2 according to the pulse ox)?

**Mechanical issues
(lead fell off, tube is blocked, O_2 is not connected)**

If a neonate has been treated with antibiotics, what vitamin deficiency is he or she at some risk to develop?

Vitamin K
(poor absorption & decreased synthesis in the gut)

When can "fortifier" be added to breast milk for preterm infants?

After the second week of life
(Fortifier adds calcium, phos, iron, & vitamin D)

How should iron be provided to preterm infants on TPN?
(type & amount)

- Elemental iron
- 2 mg/kg/day

When should iron supplementation of TPN begin, for premature infants?

1–2 months after birth

What three organ systems should you consider when diagnosing the cause of cyanosis in a newborn (or anyone, for that matter)?

Cardiovascular
Pulmonary
Central nervous system

What causes respiratory distress syndrome (RDS) in newborns?

Lack of surfactant

In a normal pregnancy, when is surfactant produced, and which cells produce it?

- **After 32 weeks**
- **Type II alveolar cells (aka pneumocytes)**

If early delivery is anticipated, what medication can you give to the mother to accelerate surfactant production?

Steroids!

In general, what naturally occurring situations hasten surfactant production?

Fetal stressors
(such as maternal hypertension, narcotic addiction, premature rupture of membranes, IUGR, and sickle cell disease)

What is the typical course of neonatal RDS?

Develops in first hours
Worsens for 2–3 days
Improves

A hallmark of recovery from RDS is what secondary effect?

"Brisk" diuresis

The classic appearance of an RDS chest X-ray is described as what sort of pattern?

Reticulogranular
(Heart border may be lost)

Prematurity is, of course, a risk factor for RDS. What are the five other known risk factors?
(1 maternal)
(1 family history)
(3 current birth history)

1. Maternal diabetes
2. Previous infant with RDS
3. Perinatal asphyxia
4. Second twin
5. C-section delivery

What percentage of infants born <30 weeks will develop RDS without treatment?

60 %
(Drops to 35 % if steroids are given)

If antenatal steroids are given, how long is their positive effect on pulmonary maturity known to last, and when does the effect begin?

Effect begins 24 h after dosing –
Lasts at least 7 days
(data not available beyond 7 days, so when re-dosing for later bouts of preterm labor is needed is not clear)

Surfactant therapy is available for infants who cannot produce adequate quantities. What are the two types of surfactant treatment?

- "Rescue" treatment after RDS begins
- "Prophylactic" treatment at delivery

Which infants are the best candidates for prophylactic surfactant therapy?

<26 weeks

What two treatment modalities are available for RDS?

Surfactant
&
Supportive care

A variety of problems may lead to persistent pulmonary hypertension (PPHN). What is the overall prognosis?

**Good –
<10 % mortality**

How quickly does PPHN present?

**Quickly –
During the first day of life**

Which newborns are most at risk for PPHN, in terms of gestational age?

Term or Postterm infants!

What two aspects of the birth history tell you that the infant is at increased risk for PPHN?

Low Apgars
&
C-section delivery

The cause of PPHN is often idiopathic. What two anatomical problems are known to cause or contribute to PPHN?

Pulmonary hypoplasia
&
Congenital diaphragmatic hernia

What sort of lung disease seems to contribute to the development of PPHN?

Interstitial lung disease
(pneumonia, meconium aspiration)

Why would acidosis & hypoxemia contribute to the development of PPHN?

Both cause vasoconstriction in the pulmonary vessels (increasing pressure)

Newborns with what hematological condition are at increased risk for PPHN?

Hyperviscosity
(usually due to polycythemia)

In PPHN, is the heart structurally normal?

Generally, yes

If a newborn with PPHN is given supplemental O_2 (oxygen challenge test), what will the result be?

Postductal F_iO_2 will improve

Why would too much pressure in the pulmonary artery lead to a low O_2 anyway?

The pressure causes right to left shunting over the PDA or foramen ovale

What therapies are helpful in reducing right to left cardiac shunting, for PPHN patients? (3 main ones)

Inhaled nitric oxide
Volume expansion
&
Inotropes (increases left sided pressure)

In very severe & unstable cases of PPHN, what invasive technique can be used as a temporizing measure?

ECMO
(extra-corporeal membrane oxygenation)

What are the mainstays of PPHN treatment?
(1 activity-based)
(1 hematological)
(1 acid–base)
(2 medications)

1. **Minimize exertion/stress -provide sedation, minimal stimulation**
2. **Maintain a good hematocrit**
3. **Induce normal to slightly elevated pH (pH 7.40 target)**
4. **Nitric oxide (dilates pulmonary vessels)**
5. **Broad spectrum antibiotics**

For a PPHN patient on 100 % O_2 what is the typical PaO_2 (measured at a postductal site)?

About 40

How can you differentiate PPHN from structural heart disease? (2 ways)

Cardiac evaluations are normal (exam, chest X-ray, echo)
&
Supplemental O_2 improves PaO_2 (>100–150) in PPHN, but has little effect on most structural cardiac problems (the exception being TAPVR)

What is the usual pathophysiology of ROP (retinopathy of prematurity)? (3 steps)

1. High concentration of $O_2 \rightarrow$ retinal vasoconstriction
2. Retinal capillaries are damaged
3. Retinal vessels proliferate, in response

Which neonates are <u>always</u> at risk to develop ROP?

<30 weeks gestation
  Or
<1,300 g
(even without supplemental oxygen exposure)

If an infant has known ROP, how often should ophthalmology evaluate his/her retinas?

Every 1–2 weeks
(depending on severity)

What does "plus disease" of ROP refer to?

Tortuous & engorged blood vessels near the optic disk

When can frequent ophtho evaluations of ROP retinas be discontinued?

When the retina is fully vascularized

When necessary, how is retinopathy of prematurity treated?

Laser therapy
(if untreated, 50 % will develop blindness if laser was indicated)

As increasing amounts of fibroproliferative matter forms on the retina in ROP, what mechanical problem can develop in the retina?

Retinal detachment (stage 4 disease)

Is aortic stenosis more common in males or females?	**Males (4:1)**
How common is it to have other cardiac anomalies associated with aortic stenosis?	**Common (20 %)**
What other cardiac problems are associated with aortic stenosis? (4)	**1. Coarctation** **2. PDA** **3. Bicuspid valve** **4. Left heart obstructive lesions (e.g., hypoplastic left heart)**
How is aortic stenosis typically corrected? (two methods)	Catheter-based expansion Or Valve replacement
What infection must you always watch for with cardiac valve disease (general category)?	Subacute bacterial endocarditis
What determines the severity of symptoms from aortic stenosis?	Degree of obstruction
What is the relationship between the age of presentation, and the severity of aortic stenosis?	The younger the presentation, the worse the stenosis
Severe cases of aortic stenosis are associated with which antenatal problem?	**"Non-immune" hydrops fetalis (meaning, destruction of RBCs that was not related to ABO incompatibility)**
What are typical finding of severe aortic stenosis?	**1. Cardiomegaly** **2. Hypotension** **3. Pulmonary edema/tachypnea/ respiratory distress**
Is aortic stenosis a risk factor for cardiac ischemia and infarct?	Yes – There may not be enough pressure at the aorta to "back fill" the coronary arteries

If a newborn has "critical aortic stenosis," systemic blood flow will depend on what structure?

The ductus
(must keep it open until the stenosis is surgically corrected)

What medication can be used to maintain a patent ductus arteriosus?

Prostaglandin E₂

What medication can be used to *close* a PDA?

**NSAIDs
(indomethacin, ibuprofen)**

On heart exam, would you detect a murmur with aortic stenosis? If so, where?

- **Yes**
- **The base of the heart (murmurs are heard *opposite* the direction of blood flow, in many cases)**

Where will an aortic stenosis murmur (classically) radiate to?

**The neck
(Bilateral carotids)**

Why might the murmur of aortic stenosis be absent in patients with critical stenosis?

So little blood outflow that you can't hear the flow

What is "mixed" apnea?

Central & obstructive apnea occurring together

What percentage of premature infants have apnea?

>50 %

Pathological apnea in full-term infants is usually associated with what other problem?

**GE reflux
(gastroesophageal)**

What is the classic periodic breathing pattern?

- 3 or more central apneas
- Lasting 3 s
- Occuring in a 20-s period

What are the typical physical findings associated with obstructive apnea in infants?

1. Micrognathia (small chin)
2. Macroglossia (big tongue)
3. Choanal atresia or stenosis
4. Nasal congestion/foreign body

How is anemia related to apnea?	Certain genetic & familial disorders are associated with both (such as Werdnig-Hoffman & Familial dysautonomia)
What radiographic tests might you want to obtain for an apnea patient?	• Chest X-ray (r/o pneumonia) • Lateral neck (r/o obstructive causes) • Head CT (r/o bleed)
What is the natural course for apnea of prematurity?	**Spontaneous resolution by 4 weeks post-gestational age**
Is supplemental O$_2$ useful for central apnea?	**Yes –** **Especially if the child is desaturating (minimizes hypoxia)**
Is supplemental O$_2$ useful for obstructive apnea?	Yes
What medications are useful for apnea of prematurity?	**Caffeine** **Theophylline** **(both require loading, then maintenance doses, & levels)**
Is home monitoring helpful in prevention of SIDS?	No – It is still sometimes used, but there is no proven benefit
Does a PFO (patent foramen ovale) require surgical correction?	**No –** **No significant shunt**
Do atrial septal defects cause problems in infants?	**No –** **Generally even large defects are initially asymptomatic**
What is balanitis?	**Inflammation of the tip of the penis (glans) and foreskin**
What is posthitis?	**Inflammation of the mucous membrane surface of the prepuce (doesn't involve the body of the penis)**

**What are the typical causes
of balanoposthitis?**

1. **Infection
   (anaerobes, yeast, skin flora)**
2. **Irritation
   (diapers, smegma, soap)**
3. **Trauma**

What cause of balanoposthitis must you
especially watch for in young infants?

Hair tourniquet on the penis

When should circumcision be considered
after balanitis?

1. When edema has resolved
2. If the infection or problem occurs
   more than once

Why are infants at special risk
for botulinum poisoning?

The intestinal flora of infants
is different –
Colonization is easier

How does botulinum toxin work?

**It prevents ACh release
in peripheral neuron terminals
permanently**

How is it possible for people to recover
after botulinum poisoning?

The peripheral neurons and nerve
terminals *slowly* regenerate

Infant botulism is most commonly seen
in what age range?

<6 months
(95 % are in this age range)

The typical botulinum toxin infant has
what demographics?

White
Middle-class
Breast fed
(Most often from California,
Pennsylvania, or Utah)

**What is the most common food
responsible for infant botulism?**

Honey

**What is the prognosis for appropriately
treated infant botulism?**

Excellent

The first symptoms of infant
botulism are…?
(two symptoms)

Poor feeding
    &
Constipation

**What is the pattern of paralysis
in botulism?**

**Descending –
Bulbar muscles are affected first**

What are the pupillary findings in botulism?	Mid-position & weakly reactive Or Fixed & dilated
If a patient is suspected to have botulinum toxicity, what should be sent to the state health department?	Stool sample & Food sample (if any particular food is suspected)
Why must possible botulinum samples be packaged so carefully?	Inhaled or ingested minute quantities can make workers ill
In addition to respiratory failure, what three other significant complications of botulinum poison are often seen in infants?	• Dehydration (poor feeding) • Aspiration pneumonia (airway protection lost) • Constipation & urinary retention
Is botulinum antitoxin recommended for infant botulism?	No – It is horse-serum derived, so there are lots of complications (It is recommended for older kids & adults, though)
When should you expect infant botulism to begin to improve?	2–5 weeks after presentation (a long time!)
In addition to assaying for botulinum toxin, what other test is helpful to confirm the diagnosis?	EMG
Fever, irritability, & nipple discharge or breast swelling in a neonate suggests what diagnosis?	Breast abscess/mastitis
What are the risk factors for breast abscess/mastitis in newborns? (2)	Breast hypertrophy at birth & Female gender (2:1 ratio)
What are the complications of neonatal breast abscess?	Bad stuff – Sepsis/bacteremia Cellulitis Necrotizing fasciitis Scarring of mammary gland

What are the important pathogens in neonatal mastitis or abscess?	Staph aureus is most common – E. Coli, Group B Strep, and Pseudomonas are also possible
How is uncomplicated breast abscess of the newborn treated?	• **I & D** • **IV oxacillin +/− aminoglycoside** • **14 days oral antibiotics after improvement on IV**
Should a mother breast feed from a breast affected by mastitis or abscess?	Yes, if possible – If the area is too tender, breast pumping may help
How common is thrush in healthy newborns?	**30–40 %!!!**
What are the typical complications of thrush?	**Anorexia/poor feeding**
If thrush is recurrent, what two possibilities should you consider?	• **Abnormal immune system** • **Re-inoculation (from nipples, pacifiers, toys)**
How can items be cleansed of possible yeast contamination?	**Boil for 5 min**
How is oral thrush treated? (3 options)	1. Remove plaques after each feeding 2. Optional Nystatin suspension (1–2 cc's to each cheek after feeds) 3. Ketoconazole/fluconazole if immunocompromised
Should Gentian violet be used to treat oral candidiasis?	No (It was used, at one time, for thrush – that's where this item comes from)
An infant who suddenly develops congestive heart failure, with decreased femoral pulses, in the neonatal period could have what common cardiac anomaly? *(common vignette to see on the boards!)*	**Aortic coarctation (the ductus closed)**

What is the most critical initial intervention for a neonate with coarctation who suddenly develops CHF?

Prostaglandin (E_2) infusion to open the ductus

What medications are typically used to manage CHF due to aortic coarctation?

The usual ones –
Digoxin to increase contraction strength
Furosemide to manage fluid

What metabolic derangement is most common in aortic coarctation patients who suddenly decompensate?

Acidosis –
Needs to be corrected quickly, and definitely before surgery

Is the solution for critical aortic coarctation medical or surgical?

Surgical

What are the three general reasons for congenital hypothyroidism?

1. Thyroid gland malformation
2. Hormone is made, but it's defective
3. Transient causes (maternal medications, iodine exposure, maternal antibodies)

How common is congenital hypothyroidism?

**Common –
1 per 3,000–4,000 births
(US and worldwide)**

Defective thyroid hormone synthesis is inherited. What is the inheritance pattern?

Autosomal recessive
(at least 15 different defects are known)

Are defects in thyroid gland formation or thyroid hormone synthesis more common?

Gland formation –
80 % of cases

How long do you have to begin treatment for hypothyroidism, in order to prevent permanent damage?

4 weeks!

Vasospasm is most often associated with use of what type of catheter?

Umbilical artery catheters

What is the treatment of choice for vasospasm associated with an arterial catheter?

Removal
(if feasible)

How would you notice a catheter-related vasospasm on physical exam?

A limb turns white or blue

In addition to vasospasm (contraction) of the vessel, what other catheter-related problems could cause white or blue color change in a limb?

Thrombus or embolus

Complete loss of pulses in an affected white or blue limb suggests what possible arterial catheter-related event?

Thrombus

How can you diagnose thrombosis in the neonate?
(two ways)

Ultrasound
(preferably with Doppler color flow imaging)
   Or
Angiogram

When should you <u>not remove</u> the catheter, even though you suspect vasospasm?
(3 situations)

1. Thrombosis is suspected
2. The catheter is critical to care
3. Spasm is mild

What is the general idea behind conservative treatment for vasospasm in the lower extremities?

Vasodilate the <u>unaffected</u> leg –
This causes reflex dilation in the opposite extremity, relieving the vascular spasm

Aggressive treatment of vasospasm (short of removing the catheter) centers on infusion of what two substances?

Tolazoline
   &
Papaverine
(both vasodilators)

Can ischemia follow episodes of vasospasm (even after resolution)?

Yes

How is catheter-associated *thrombosis* treated?
(2 ways)

Consult vascular surgery
for possible immediate removal
   Or
Streptokinase
(thrombolytics)

ABO incompatibility is responsible for what fraction of hemolytic disease in newborns?

2/3

Symptomatic ABO incompatibility occurs most commonly for mothers with what specific blood type?

Type O (both Rh + and −)
(More IgG is produced by Type O mothers. IgM predominates in Types A & B, which is too big to cross the placenta)

What antibodies are responsible for ABO incompatibility/anemia in newborns?

Maternal IgG

How is anemia defined for a full-term infant?

<13
(50 % is fetal Hgb also known as HgbF)

Does ABO incompatibility typically produce a severe anemia?

**No –
Not even in subsequent pregnancies**
(There are various reasons for this – fetal cells have fewer A or B antigen sites, other organ tissues have quite a lot for antibodies to bind to, and most maternal A & B antibodies are IgM so they don't cross the placenta)

What clinical sign of ABO incompatibility hemolysis is typically seen?

Early (first 24 h) & rapidly evolving jaundice

How is ABO incompatibility hemolysis of the newborn treated (if treatment is needed)?

Phototherapy (rising bilirubin)
    Or
Exchange transfusion if severe

"Microspherocytes" on peripheral blood smear are a buzzword for which type of neonatal anemia?

**ABO incompatibility
(*not* generally seen with Rh incompatibility)**

What common blood incompatibility does produce moderate to severe anemia?

Rh incompatibility

Why is Rh incompatibility so much more destructive to fetal RBCs than ABO incompatibility?
(3 reasons)

1. Rh antigen is only found on RBCs and not other tissue sites
2. Fetal RBCs have a lot more Rh antigen versus A or B antigen sites
3. Rh antibodies are usually IgG, so they easily cross the placental barrier

Ninety-percent of Rh-based hemolytic disease is due to which type of Rh antigen?

D
(the remainder are usually due to C or E)

Are there other blood incompatibilities, in addition to Rh D, that frequently cause significant hemolysis?

Yes –
Rh antigens:Anti-C, Anti-c (small "c"), Anti-E
Minor groups: Fya (Duffy), Kell, and Kidd groups

Rh immunoglobulin (RhoGam®) contains immunoglobulin to which Rh antigen?

D

Rh- mothers who are not treated with RhoGam® develop Rh antibodies about 15 % of the time. RhoGam treatment has lowered this number to what percent?

1 %

In addition to anemia, what are the main presenting signs of Rh incompatibility anemia?

1. **Jaundice**
2. **Hepatosplenomegaly (clearance sites for RBCs & reticulocyte formation)**
3. **Hydrops fetalis**

What is hydrops fetalis?

Fetal edema with profound anemia

Why are erythroblastosis fetalis babies (those affected by Rh incompatibility producing anemia) not usually jaundiced at birth, despite having a lot of hemolysis?

The bilirubin crosses the placenta – Mom's body processes it
(so neither mom nor baby are jaundiced when the baby is born)

Will erythroblastosis fetalis babies become jaundiced after birth?

Yes –
Usually quickly
(that's why jaundice is one of the presenting signs, even though it's not present at birth)

What special birth injury are erythro-blastosis fetalis babies at special risk for?

Splenic rupture

Why would erythroblastosis fetalis patients be pancytopenic at birth, in some cases?

The pluripotent blood stem cells were all busy trying to make enough RBCs, and they failed to make other cell lines!

Why are erythroblastosis fetalis infants at risk for hypoglycemia?

Circulating hemoglobin interferes with insulin –
Islet cells increase in response, producing hyperinsulinemia!!!

If an Rh- mother received Rh immunoglobulin at 28-weeks or later (as she should), what will a "direct Coombs test" of the baby's blood show?

It will be (falsely) positive!
Reminder:
The direct Coombs directly looks for attacking antibodies. IgG in the mother will cross to the fetus – even if we inject it

How can you tell when the direct Coombs test is falsely positive, due to RhoGam administration?

The infant has no reticulocytosis – the dose is too small to cause any response

How are fetuses of mothers with known Rh antibodies evaluated?
(two ways)

Ultrasound –
Looks for evidence of hydrops fetalis
    &
Amniocentesis –
Looks for elevated bili level in the amniotic fluid

What are the two mainstays of treatment for moderate to severe Rh incompatible anemia?

Exchange transfusion
    &
Phototherapy
(useful to decrease the number of transfusions needed)

What are the fluids of choice for resuscitating a neonate with hydrops fetalis?

O negative blood
    &
Fresh frozen plasma

What are the two main features of hydrops fetalis?

Edema (generalized)
    &
Severe anemia

If a fetus has severe anemia, what related problems is this likely to generate?

- High output cardiac failure
- Hypoxemia & acidosis

Part of the reason infants with hydrops fetalis are so edematous, is the low protein content of their blood. What other fluid collections often develop in this setting?

Ascites
&
Pleural effusions

Rh incompatibility is most likely in which ethnic group? Most unlikely group?

- Caucasians (15 %)
- Asians (approximately 0)
  *(African Americans have
  a frequency of 7 %)*

In general, hemolytic anemias cause elevation in indirect (unconjugated) bilirubin. Severe Rh can also cause elevated *direct* bilirubin. How?

The large amount of hematopoeisis in the liver can obstruct the canaliculi
(typically at 5–6 days after birth)

How do you follow the severity of a hemolytic anemia in a neonate?

Serial bilirubins

Schistocytes or helmet cells are associated with which type of anemias?

**Consumption anemia
(microangiopathic anemia)**

If transfusion is needed at birth, what is the target hematocrit for the ingoing blood?

**50 %
(higher than usual!)**

Can blood drawn from a placental vein be used for transfusion?

**Yes –
If it is heparinized & filtered**

What is the maximum cc's per kilogram that can be transfused in a single episode (unless central venous pressure is directly monitored)?

10 cc's per kg

In what situation is iron supplementation helpful for neonatal anemia?
(3)

1. Preterm infant
2. Fetal-maternal hemorrhage
3. Chronic twin-twin transfusion (one twin stealing blood supply from the other)

Erythropoeitin can be given to decrease the need for transfusions after what age?

2–3 weeks old

There are two types of neonatal thrombocytopenia. What are they?	**Isoimmune** **(from mother's antibodies)** **&** **Autoimmune** **(from the child's own antibodies)**
In a case of isoimmune thrombocytopenia, what replacement platelets should be given if the count is very low (<20,000)?	<u>Maternal</u> platelets (her antibody won't attack her own cells)
What hematocrit defines polycythemia *in the newborn?*	Central venous hematocrit of ≥65
Why is 65 the critical hematocrit value for polycythemia in the newborn?	**Blood viscosity rises exponentially beginning at a hematocrit of 65**
Do all infants with hematocrits of 65 or greater develop symptoms of hyperviscosity?	**No**
Do infants with hematocrits below 65 sometimes develop hyperviscosity syndrome?	**Yes**
How are neonates somewhat protected from hyperviscosity despite their high hematocrits?	Their fibrinogen level is low (This decreases plasma viscosity and also RBC aggregation)
Why do in utero endocrine disorders contribute to polycythemia?	They increase oxygen demand (stimulating formation of more RBCs)
Why is Beckwith-Wiedemann syndrome associated with polycythemia in the neonate?	**Secondary hyperinsulinism** **(It's part of the syndrome, and it increases RBC formation)**
What three typical trisomies are associated with polycythemia?	**13, 18, & 21**
How does placental "hypertransfusion" contribute to polycythemia?	If a larger than usual amount of blood enters the infant's circulation, fluid shifts may → polycythemia

Why would intrapartum asphyxia (not chronic, in this case) contribute to polycythemia?

Fetal distress increases umbilical blood flow toward the fetus (Acidosis will also encourage fluid shifts out of the intravascular space, increasing the hematocrit further)

What is the most appropriate management for an infant with asymptomatic polycythemia?

Observation

What is the main way that neonatal polycythemia causes long-term problems?

Damage to the CNS – Usually multiple subtle problems

What is the utility of a partial exchange transfusion (PET) in the treatment of polycythemia?

- It may or may not decrease neurological sequelae (reports are mixed – most say not effective)
- It increases NEC and other GI disorders

(PET is the main treatment modality)

What *is* a partial exchange transfusion?

Some blood is phlebotomized out of the circulation, and replaced with saline to lower the hematocrit

Why is PET used at all, in the treatment of polycythemia?

It decreases acute, though usually not long-term, problems

Are too many RBCs the cause of thrombotic problems in polycythemia?

No – It is multifactorial. Not the number of RBCs alone (Factors involved are not yet clear)

What is the most common hematological abnormality seen in newborns admitted to the NICU?

Thrombocytopenia (due to increased platelet destruction)

What are the causes, in general, of newborn thrombocytopenia? (3 general categories)

1. Maternal causes (drugs, infectious, autoimmune disease, coagulopathies)
2. Placental disorders
3. Neonatal causes (drugs, infections, congenital syndromes, giant hemangioma, metabolic disorders)

Thrombocytopenia co-occurs with physical malformations or abnormalities in what four cases?	1. Trisomy syndromes 2. Giant hemangioma (Kassabach-Merit syndrome) 3. *Rubella syndrome* 4. Thrombocytopenia – Absent radius syndrome (TAR)
How does the size of the platelet help you to know the underlying cause of thrombo-cytopenia? (meaning decreased production vs. increased destruction)	Large – destruction Normal size – Decreased production
If rapid platelet destruction is the problem, what will happen when you give a platelet transfusion?	Little or no increase in platelet count
If a fetus is known to have significant thrombocytopenia, is vaginal delivery an option?	No – Platelets of <100,000 gives a significant risk of intracerebral hemorrhage during birth
When is a platelet transfusion indicated for a neonate?	**1. Active bleeding** **2. Platelet count <20,000**
What quantity of platelets should be transfused for a neonate?	**10–20 cm³/kg**
When random donor platelets are given to a thrombocytopenic neonate, in what ways should they be matched to the baby's blood?	ABO & Rh
Why do premature infants have a more profound "anemia of infancy" than full-term infants? (4)	1. Fewer RBCs made by time of birth 2. Shorter RBC lifespan 3. More rapid body growth 4. Lower erythropoietin
If the umbilical cord is occluded during delivery, the infant will be missing about how much of the blood supply (in cc's)?	30 cc's

What are the typical causes   **Nuchal cord**
of umbilical cord occlusion?   **Or**
                   (2)   **Prolapsed cord**

What complication   **Nondepressed linear skull fracture**
(not usually requiring treatment)   **– 5 %**
sometimes occurs with
cephalohematoma?

Cephalohematoma is associated with what   Primiparity
two risk factors?   &
                                             Vacuum extraction

Congenital thrombocytopenia is associated   The radii
with absence of what bone in a particular
congenital syndrome?

What metabolic enzyme deficiencies   1. G6PD deficiency
sometimes cause neonatal anemia?   2. Pyruvate kinase deficiency
                   (2)

If thalassemia presents as anemia   **Homozygous alpha-thalassemia**
at birth, what type of thalassemia
are you dealing with?

Will the pallor of acute or chronic   **No**
hemorrhagic anemia improve with
supplemental O$_2$?

How high must the unsaturated hemo-   **>5**
globin be to produce cyanosis?

Hemolytic anemias typically present with   Jaundice
what physical finding?   (The compensatory reticulocytosis
                                             may keep the hemoglobin within
                                             normal limits, initially)

What is the characteristic presentation   1. No jaundice
of hypoplastic anemia in the neonate?   2. No reticulocyte response
                   (3)   3. Presents after 48 h old

Which neonatal anemias typically cause   • Those that develop relatively
hepatosplenomegaly, in general terms?   slowly
                                             • Those with reticulocyte response

Normocytic/normochromic anemia suggests what causes for the neonatal anemia?

(4)

1. Acute hemorrhage
2. Hypoplastic anemia
3. Intrinsic RBC defect
4. General, systemic, disease

How do you calculate the "corrected reticulocyte count?"
(adjusts for the hematocrit)

$$\frac{\text{Observed retics} \times \text{observed Hct}}{\text{Normal hematocrit}}$$

Neonates with a microcytic/hypochromic anemia are likely to have what three underlying problems?

1. Twin-twin transfusion
2. Fetomaternal hemorrhage
3. Alpha-thalassemia
(Hypochromic means the patient is losing, or not using, iron)

Elliptocytes on peripheral blood smear suggest with "zebra" diagnosis?

Hereditary elliptocytosis
(at least they named it well!)

"Pyknocytes" on the peripheral blood smear indicate what cause of neonatal anemia?

G6PD deficiency

Neonates who are anemic, and also have ongoing difficulties with apnea, are likely to benefit from what treatment?

Transfusion
(better O_2 capacity can be helpful – continuous monitoring data supports it)

Persistent (>24 h) tachycardia or poor weight gain in an anemic neonate suggests what treatment may be needed?

Transfusion
(to improve O_2 capacity)

Vitamin E is given to prevent anemia in which neonatal patient population?

Preemies
(unless they are breast fed)

Which infants are likely to need folate supplementation?
(3 groups)

1. Preemies or low birth weight infants
2. Dilantin patients
3. Those with increased erythropoeisis

What are the two main causes of "consumptive coagulopathy" in neonates?

Bacterial & viral infections
(including congenital ones)
&
Thromboplastin embolism

How is severe anemia due to consumptive coagulopathy treated?
(3 ways)

- Treat the underlying cause
- Exchange transfusion
- FFP or platelets (controversial)

How might a neonate be exposed to a thromboplastin embolus?

Through disorders involving tissue necrosis
(NEC, dead twin in utero, maternal toxemia, etc.)

Why might a neonate present with acute hemorrhagic anemia more than 24-h after birth, if vitamin K was given properly?

Occult obstetrical trauma – usually to solid organs
(Liver is most common)

What is the most common "multiple congenital anomaly" syndrome?

Down's
(Trisomy 21)

How common is Down syndrome?

Very common –
1:600 live births

What two serious malformations sometimes accompany Down syndrome?

Heart defects
(especially of the center of the heart)
&
GI atresia/imperforate anus

Why are Down syndrome infants at greater risk for aspiration and difficulty breathing?

Hypotonia
(affects the bulbar muscles, as well as the other muscles)

What are some typical physical findings/ characteristics for Down's syndrome infants?
(1 muscle)
(2 facial)
(2 hand)

1. Hypotonia
2. Slanted eyes with epicanthal fold, hypertelorism (wide-set eyes)
3. Single palmar crease & short 5th digit that curve inward

What is the other name for Trisomy 18?

Edwards' syndrome

In addition to Down syndrome, what other chromosomal disorders are most commonly diagnosed?

Turner syndrome (45, X)
Trisomy 18 (Edwards)
Trisomy 13 (Patau)

**What are the typical characteristics
of Trisomy 18 babies?**
(5)

1. **IUGR**
2. **Micrognathia**
3. *Congenital heart disease (95 %!)*
4. *Hypertonic muscles*
5. **"Rocker-bottom" club feet**

What three facial abnormalities
are typical for Trisomy 18?

- Micrognathia (small chin)
- Ptosis
- Abnormal ears

**What hand abnormality goes
with Trisomy 18?**

"Overlapping" digits

**What chest abnormality goes
with Trisomy 18?**

Short sternum

**What is the prognosis for Trisomy 18
infants?**

Only 10 % survive to 1 year old
(most die in the first 3 months)

**What is the prognosis for Trisomy 13
(Patau's)?**

**Almost always lethal in the first
3 months**

**How common is congenital heart
disease in Trisomy 13 (Patau's)?**

>95 %

**Which common multiple congenital
anomaly syndrome is associated with
cystic kidneys and a hooked penis?**

**Trisomy 13
(Patau's)**

What craniofacial abnormalities go
with Trisomy 13 (Patau's)?
(4)

1. Cleft lip/
   palate +/−holoprosencephaly
2. Cutis aplasia of the scalp
3. Microphthalmos
4. Bulbous nose

**"Rockerbottom" clubfeet combined
with polydactyly suggests what common
multiple congenital anomaly syndrome?**

**Patau's
(Trisomy 13)**

**What percentage of Turner syndrome
fetuses are stillborn or spontaneously
miscarry?**

95 %

What cardiac anomaly is especially common with Turner syndrome?

Aortic coarctation

What chest abnormality is commonly noted in Turner syndrome?

Shield chest

What physical findings are considered to be typical for Turner syndrome?
(2 neck)
(1 habitus)
(1 foot finding)

1. **Webbed neck & nuchal edema**
2. **Short stature**
3. **Pedal edema**

What neck finding is typically seen in Down syndrome?

Redundant skin at nape of neck
(can often be seen on fetal US, also)

"Potter's oligohydramnios sequence" is a multiple congenital anomalies (MCA) syndrome second only to what other MCA in frequency?

Down syndrome
(1:600 live births for Down
1:4,000 live births for Potter)

What is the prognosis for the oligohydramnios sequence infant?

Bad –
Virtually all die
A new experimental treatment using saline to replace the missing amniotic fluid may change the prognosis! This material is too new, though, to be on the board exam

What is the pathophysiology of Potter's syndrome?

Renal agenesis → oligohydramnios (inadequate production of amniotic fluid) → pulmonary hypoplasia

What is the risk of recurrence in future pregnancies, if one fetus has oligohydramnios sequence?

2–7 %
(depends on the specific cause)

Why do oligohydramnios infants sometimes have "prune bellies?"

Sometimes the kidneys were initially hydronephrotic, which stretched the belly
(then the kidneys atrophied, leaving the belly empty)

Why can amniotic band syndrome be especially difficult to diagnose?

In 90 % of the cases, the bands are gone before delivery
(The malformations sometimes suggest another syndrome initially)

What two types of effects occur in amniotic band syndrome?

Biomechanical deformities (mainly altered limbs & digits)
&
Viscera unable to return to the abdomen/ectopia cordis

Do all amniotic bands cause malformations?

No –
Those not attached to the fetus do not seem to

In cases of amniotic band syndrome, what findings are often observed with inspection of the amnion?
(3 possibilities)

- Small amnion
- Absent amnion
- Amnion rolled into strands

What does arthrogryposis refer to?

Multiple joint "fixations" (joint extensions, contractures, and dislocations)

In about 90 % of cases, how does arthrogryposis develop?

Brain or spinal cord abnormalities →
Fetal inactivity →
Abnormal fetal joint development

What craniofacial abnormalities are common in amniotic band syndrome?

Encephalocele
    &
Facial clefts

How is arthrogryposis managed?

Physical therapy/rehab
    &
Ortho consultation early

How does Pierre Robin syndrome develop?

Severe mandibular hypoplasia →
Glossoptosis →
Upper airway obstruction +
cleft palate

What is glossoptosis?

Bunched up tongue (not enough space for it stretch out, because the mandible is so small)

What are the three main craniofacial features of Pierre Robin?

- Micrognathia
- Cleft palate
- Low-set ears

Do infants with Pierre Robin have associated malformations of other organs in some cases?

No –
If other malformations are found, it is probably a syndrome
(Pierre Robin is a sequence)

What is the risk of recurrence for future pregnancies if one infant is born with Pierre Robin?

**Unrelated –
It's not an inherited disorder**

How is Pierre Robin managed in the long-term?

The mandible grows out in time, correcting the problem

What are the two main problems for Pierre Robin sequence infants?

Airway distress
&
Difficulty feeding

How are Pierre Robin respiratory difficulties treated in mild cases?

Prone position with head <u>lower</u> than body

How are moderate & severe cases of Pierre Robin treated, in terms of respiratory distress?
(3)

1. Oral obturators will sometimes work
2. Temporary suture fixation of the tongue is sometimes performed
3. Tracheostomy (until the mandible grows)

What is the distinction between a congenital "syndrome" and a congenital "sequence?"

Sequence – multiple effects follow from a single malformation

**(physical or mechanical abnormality)
Syndrome – multiple effects result from the same genetic error**

How is an "association" different from a syndrome or sequence of congenital anomalies?

"Associations" are collections of congenital anomalies not usually due to a single genetic or biomechanical cause

What is the "VATER" association of congenital anomalies?

Vertebral anomalies
Anal atresia
Tracheo-esophageal fistula
Esophageal atresia
Radial defects

VATER association infants sometimes also have what four additional problems?

Cardiac defects
Renal defects
Small intestine atresia
Hydrocephalus

VATER is a common associate (1:5,000 live births). CHARGE association is less common, but often more life threatening. What is the CHARGE association?

Coloboma (iris & retinal cleft)
Heart defects
Atresia – choanal
Retarded growth/development
Genital anomalies
Ear defects/deafness

In addition to potentially life threatening heart defects and choanal atresia, what other life threatening problem may CHARGE newborns exhibit?

Profound difficulties with swallowing

For any newborn with respiratory distress, and no clear etiology, what simple test to rule-out a mechanical problem should be performed?

Pass an NG into each nare to rule-out choanal atresia or stenosis

Cardiac problems (usually conotruncal), + small abnormal ears, + mild facial dysmorphology in a newborn should suggest what diagnosis?

DiGeorge syndrome
(there is usually some mention of calcium troubles to help you)

What lab abnormalities suggest a DiGeorge syndrome diagnosis?

Hypocalcemia +/– low lymphocyte count

Why do DiGeorge syndrome infants have low lymphocyte counts?

Partial or total lack of thymic development

Why do DiGeorge syndrome patients develop hypocalcemia?

Missing or hypoplastic parathyroid development

Velocardiofacial syndrome and DiGeorge syndrome are very similar. How are they different?

Velocardiofacial has cleft palate & a more unusual facial appearance

What is the genetic error that usually produces DiGeorge & velocardiofacial syndrome?

22q11 region deletion

What is the other name for lethal skeletal dysplasias?

Lethal short-limb, short-rib dwarfism

What is the general etiology of lethal skeletal dysplasias?

All are genetic disorders

Skeletal disproportion in an infant with respiratory distress suggests what diagnosis?

A type of lethal short-limb, short-rib dwarfism

What diagnostics should be completed ASAP if a lethal skeletal dysplasia is suspected? Why?

- Babygram X-ray
- Prognosis & risk of recurrence depend on specific diagnosis

If lethal skeletal dysplasia is suspected, what two things do you look for on the babygram X-ray?

Small chest
&
Long bone abnormalities

Refractory hypoglycemia in a neonate should suggest what diagnosis?

Beckwith syndrome
(same as Beckwith-Wiedemann)

What four characteristics usually accompany Beckwith-Wiedemann syndrome?

- Macroglossia
- Gigantism
- Omphalocele
- Refractory hypoglycemia

An odd limb finding is sometimes seen with Beckwith-Wiedemann syndrome. What is it?

Unilateral limb hypertrophy

Why is it important to diagnose Beckwith-Wiedemann early?

Aggressive management of hypoglycemia prevents mental retardation

Do Beckwith-Wiedemann patients present without obvious physical findings?

Yes –
20 % will have one or zero obvious findings (but will have hypoglycemia)

Infants with fetal hydantoin syndrome have many dysmorphisms that are similar to other syndromes. What unique feature identifies them?

Missing or hypoplastic *fifth fingernails* & *toenails*

What is hypertelorism?

Wide set eyes

What are the typical facial features of fetal hydantoin syndrome? (three categories)

Eyes – epicanthal fold, ptosis, hypertelorism
Nose – Broad, flat, nasal bridge
Ears – Large & misshaped

What limb findings are sometimes seen in FAS (fetal alcohol syndrome)?

Diffusely hypoplastic nails
Mnemonic:
Alcohol affects your whole body (all of the nails), antiseizure meds are more selective (just the 5th digit nail)

Infants with FAS sometimes do not have the typical facial features. How might these children demonstrate their FAS?

Microcephaly
&
Overall small for gestational age

Internal organs are not usually affected in FAS. When they are, the organ typically affected is…?

The heart
(as usual)

Fetal isotretinoin syndrome will also occur with megadosing of what vitamin?

Vitamin A

What proportion of fetuses exposed to isotretinoin develops problems due to the exposure?

¼
(high, but not as high as all of the warnings would make you think)

When a fetus develops isotretinoin syndrome, what problems is he or she likely to develop?
(3)

1. Hydrocephalus
2. Facial abnormalities
   (various including microtia)
3. Heart defects

What is the main feature of fetal valproate syndrome?

Neural tube defects

If internal organs are affected in fetal valproate syndrome, what organ is most likely to be affected?

The heart
(as usual)

Do fetal valproate syndrome infants have limb or facial abnormalities?

Sometimes –
Limb – clubfeet & hypospadias (it's kind of a limb)
Face – various

Neural tube defects are the hallmark of what teratogenic medication's fetal syndrome?

Valproate

Diffusely hypoplastic nails goes with what common teratogenic syndrome?

FAS
(Remember: ETOH affects the whole body, anti-seizure meds are more specific – only 5th digits affected)

A neonate is born with facial abnormalities, a heart problem, and hydrocephalus. Mom has been megadosing vitamins from the "health food" store. What vitamin is likely to be responsible?

Vitamin A

What facial phenotype is associated with fetal cocaine syndrome?

**None –
The face is usually normal**

What two organ systems are most commonly affected in fetal cocaine syndrome?

CNS
  &
Genitourinary

An irritable, small for gestational age infant, with signs that look like opiate withdrawal is likely suffering from what syndrome?

Fetal cocaine syndrome

Infants of diabetic mothers are at greatest risk for what four typical malformations?

1. Sacral agenesis
2. Femoral hypoplasia
3. Heart defects
4. Cleft palate
(also associated with hypoplastic left colon)

"Tight control" of maternal diabetes can lower her infant's risk of malformation to baseline. True or false?

False –
It lowers it, but not to baseline

In general, having a mother with diabetes increases an infant's likelihood of malformation how many times?	3×
Diabetic mothers are at increased risk for children with malformations. The likelihood of malformations is most closely correlated with what diabetic parameter?	**Degree of hyperglycemia** *before* **conception** *(usually evaluated with hemoglobin A1C)*
Even with excellent glycemic management, what continues to be a problem for infants of diabetic mothers?	Macrosomia
What kind of cardiomyopathy is seen in infants of diabetic mothers, especially?	Thickening of the ventricles & septum *Usually asymptomatic & spontaneously resolves*
Infants of diabetic mothers often are large for gestational age (LGA) with hypoglycemia. What other lab abnormality is frequently seen in those neonates?	Polycythemia/elevated hematocrit (thought to be due to elevated erythropoietin)
What GI anatomical abnormality is related to maternal diabetes?	**Hypoplastic left colon Mnemonic: Large body, small Left colon**
Why does maternal diabetes increase the risk of pulmonary problems for the infant? (2 reasons)	**Insulin blocks synthesis of surfactant precursors** (mainly lectin) **& Glycogen in the lungs disrupts normal function**
Are infants of diabetic mothers at higher risk for obesity in later life, compared to those born to non-diabetic mothers?	**Yes**
Why would infants of diabetic mothers be at increased risk of hyperbilirubinemia? (2 reasons)	**Polycythemia & Increased possibility of birth trauma due to size** *(1/3 will have high bili)*

What unusual GI anomaly is associated with maternal diabetes?

Small left colon (hypoplastic or microcolon)

Which unusual vertebral abnormality is associated with maternal diabetes?

Spinal agenesis
(with "caudal regression syndrome")

How are the risks for fetuses different, depending on whether the Mom is a gestational diabetic (only), or has diabetes all the time?

Gestational diabetes does not increase congenital abnormalities or risk of future obesity & diabetes mellitus (DM does)

How common is hypoglycemia in infants of diabetic mothers?

Common – 25–50 % will develop it in the first 24 h

Why is hypocalcemia in the infant of a diabetic Mom especially concerning?

Cardiac problems – Mainly Q-T prolongation

What are you supposed to do if an infant is symptomatic with hypocalcemia?

Give 2 ml/kg 10 % calcium gluconate over 5 min

What birth complication increases the probability that the infant of a diabetic Mom will develop hypocalcemia?

Asphyxia (mechanism unclear)

What is "vanishing twin" phenomenon?

>½ of twins identified in the first trimester "disappear," leaving just one fetus in utero
(no problems seem to result)

About what proportion of twins are monozygotic in the US?

1/3

Which US ethnic group is most likely to have twins?

African Americans

Which US ethnic group is least likely to have twins?

Asians

What proportion of twins is born C-section?

½

What proportion of triplets is born C-section?

About ¾

Twin A will have a vertex presentation what percentage of the time?

80 %

When twins are born, what three structures are examined to determine the type of twinning?

- **Placenta (single, fused, or separate)**
- **Chorion**
- **Amnion**

How likely is a twin gestation to have a single amnion?

<1 %

Seventy percent of monozygotic twins have a single chorion. What is the significance of a single chorion?

The fetal circulation may commingle (mix)

Twin gestations are at increased risk for what three problems with the placental structures?

1. **Abnormal structure or insertion**
2. **More twisting/trauma**
3. **Often missing "Wharton's jelly" at the insertion site (increased risk of thrombosis)**

Are monochorionic twins monozygotic or dizygotic?

<u>Monochorionic =</u>
<u>Monozygotic</u>

Are dichorionic, same-sex twins monozygotic or dizygotic?

Can't tell without genetic studies of the infants

How would you put each group in rank order for risk of perinatal death – first-born singletons, second-born singletons, and twins (all types)?

Greatest – twins
Middle – first born singletons
Lowest – second born singletons

Of all twin types, which have the highest mortality? Why?

Monoamniotic –
Significant risk of cord tangling

For monochorionic twins, how likely is the death of one twin late in pregnancy to result in problems for the other fetus?

50 % of surviving twins will develop major complications or die

What kind of twins could be born conjoined?

Monoamniotic
(the cells can't merge unless
the cells are directly apposed)
These twins are also monochorionic,
of course

How often are conjoined twins born?

1 per 50,000
(typically the fusion is at the chest or belly)

What is the basic idea behind rates of twin mortality?

The more separate the twins are, the better

A dichorionic, diamnionic placenta usually indicates what type of twin gestation?

Fraternal

Identical twins usually have what type of chorionic membrane arrangement?

Monochorionic

Is treatment available for twin-twin transfusion?

Yes –
Laser can be used to eliminate the connection

To be sure you remember, which type of twins is at risk for twin-twin transfusion?

Monochorionic placentas –
They can commingle their blood supply

What is the perinatal mortality rate for triplets?

25 %

How often are triplet gestations born prematurely?

85 % of cases

About 50 % of twins are born with low birth weights. When does the drop-off in twin growth rates typically occur?

When their combined weight is 4 kg
(roughly the upper limit
for normal birth weight if the
pregnancy were a singleton)

Twin gestations are typically born at about how many weeks gestation?

30–34 weeks

What is the typical birthweight for a triplet?

Small –
About 1,700 g
(This is still large when you consider that $3 \times 1,700$ equals 5,100 g – large for a typical singleton or twin gestation)

What are the two main factors in twin perinatal morbidity?

Prematurity
&
Uteroplacental insufficiency

Why do monozygotic twins have 2–3 times the rate of birth defects seen in singletons & dizygotics?
(3 possible reasons)

- Space constraint → unusual biomechanical stresses
- Placental vascular anastomoses
- Increased defects in morphogenesis (NOS – not otherwise specified)

If a twin develops respiratory distress in the newborn period, is that twin likely to be the first or second born?

Second

If a twin develops necrotizing enterocolitis (NEC), is he or she likely to be the first or second born?

First-born

What social problems are especially prevalent for twins?

Child abuse
&
Inadequate nurturing

What percentage of infants with NEC were actually full-term or low-risk infants?

20 %

How is NEC thought to develop?
(3 steps)

1. **Initial ischemia or toxin injures the gut**
2. **Bacterial proliferation with enteral feeds**
3. **Gut wall invasion**

What gas produces the pockets of gas seen in pneumatosis intestinalis?

Hydrogen

What are the feared complications of NEC?

Gut necrosis, gangrene, &
perforation + peritonitis

In what way are exchange transfusions thought to contribute to NEC?

Increased variation in arterial & venous pressures during transfusion may comopromise gut blood flow

What type of feeding definitely reduces the probability of NEC developing?

Breast feeding

Polycythemia, hyperviscosity syndromes, cardiopulmonary disease with low output, and asphyxia are linked to the development of NEC due to what mechanism?

Gut ischemia/hypoxia

What is the most common early clinical sign of NEC?

Abdominal distension

What is the NEC triad of signs?

- **Abdominal distension**
- **Feeding intolerance**
- **Acute change in stool (often bloody)**

How could low-dose dopamine theoretically improve NEC?

2–4 mcg/kg/min is thought to dilate the splanchnic vascular bed

What is the typical time course for perforation relative to air in the gut wall?

Perforation usually occurs 24–48 h later

How can an umbilical vein catheter sometimes produce findings on X-ray that look like NEC?

It sometimes introduces air into the portal venous system

If NEC is diagnosed, how often should you obtain abdominal (flat plate) X-rays, and what are you watching for?

- Q 6–8 h
- Mainly free air

What radiological techniques are preferred for identification of free abdominal air in neonates?

(2)

Lateral decubitus X-ray
  Or
CT scan
(but CT is not commonly used)

What is "Stage I" NEC?

Radiology:
Normal or nonspecific

GI:
+ Residuals
+ Guaiac

Systemic:
Nonspecific changes

(lethargy, temperature changes,
bradycardia, apnea)

How is NEC organized into stages?

There are 3 components:
• Systemic symptoms
• GI problems
• Radiographic findings

NEC classification is divided into
Stage I, IIA and B, and III A & B
What is the worst one, stage IIIB?

Systemic:
Shock
Bad electrolytes

GI & Radiographic:
Perforation

Gross blood in the stool indicates
a NEC stage of at least what?

Stage IIA
(2A)

Extensive pneumatosis
intestinalis, +/− intrahepatic portal vein
gas, means what NEC stage has been
reached?

Stage IIB
(2B)

Spreading edema, erythema,
and induration of the belly is seen
in what NEC stage?

Stage IIIA
(3A)

If a NEC patient develops acidosis, he
or she is at least in what category
(stage)?

Stage IIB
(2B)

When is surgical intervention *definitely*
indicated for NEC patients?

With perforation

What are the "relative" indications for surgery in NEC patients?

1. Fixed sentinel loop >24 h (possible gangrenous bowel)
2. Deteriorating condition
3. RLQ mass
4. Abdominal wall erythema

How is spontaneous intestinal perforation in very low birth weight (VLBW) infants different from classical NEC?

Insidious onset
   &
No radiographic signs (except free air)

When VLBW infants develop spontaneous intestinal perforation, where in the gut is the perforation usually located?

Distal ileum

Are the lesions of spontaneous intestinal perforation diffuse or well localized?

Well localized

What is the prognosis for infants with spontaneous intestinal perforation?

Good
(better than with NEC)

What is the typical physical finding suggesting spontaneous intestinal perforation in VLBW infants?

Bluish discoloration of the lower abdomen
(that's an early finding)

Does NEC tend to recur?

No

What is the typical mortality of NEC with perforation?

1/3

Most NEC infants who survive are normal about 1 year later. What are the complications for the less fortunate infants? (2)

Short gut syndrome (s/p resection)
   &
Bowel obstruction (15 %)
(strictures or stenosis)

What physical finding may be present in an infant with hydrocephalus that would not be seen in an older child?

Increased head circumference
(if the fontanelles are still open)

When can cerebral ventricular dilation be a normal finding?

Ventricular dilation often precedes head growth in normal infants

What is "communicating hydrocephalus?"

The CSF passes through the base of the brain, but is blocked elsewhere

What is hydrocephalus ex vacuo?

Ventricular dilation due to loss of cerebral tissue

Obstruction in the CSF system between the 3rd ventricle and cisterna magna is which type of hydrocephalus?

Non-communicating

How is macrocephaly defined?

Head circumference ≥2 standard deviations above average (without hydrocephalus or cranial mass, of course)

What is the significance of macrocephaly without hydrocephalus?

Usually none – It's familial (sometimes related to metabolic or neuro-cutaneous diseases, or Beckwith-Weidemann syndrome)

Is excessive production of CSF a cause of hydrocephalus?

Rarely (occasionally seen with choroid plexus tumors)

What is the most common cause of hydrocephalus ex vacuo in infants?

Periventricular leukomalacia/ periventricular hemorrhage with infarct

Congenital aqueductal stenosis causes what proportion of neonatal hydrocephalus?

1/3

Congenital aqueductal stenosis is an inherited disorder. How is it inherited?

X-linked recessive (occasionally autosomal recessive)

What percentage of infants with hydrocephalus will have a breech presentation?

30 %

What percentage of infants with neural tube defects develops hydrocephalus?

Most – 80 %

If an infant has an intraventricular hemorrhage, what proportion of these infants will develop hydrocephalus?

About 1/3 –
2/3 resolve or stop expanding on their own

What three possible courses might an infant with posthemorrhagic hydrocephalus follow?

1. Spontaneous resolution or no more expansion
2. Persistent dilation
3. Rapid dilation

If possible, the course of hydrocephalus is usually observed over what period of time?

4 weeks

How reliable is papilledema as a sign of increased ICP (or hydrocephalus) in a neonate?

Not reliable

What are some typical signs of hydrocephalus developing in a neonate?
(4 findings on head exam)

1. Tense fontanelle
2. Wide skull sutures
3. Prominent scalp veins
4. Rapidly increasing head circumference

Vomiting, lethargy or irritability, apnea and bradycardia are typical general signs seen in infants with what common mechanically-based CNS problem?

Hydrocephalus

What is "setting sun sign," as related to hydrocephalus?

Sclerae are visible above the irises
(associated with developing hydrocephalus, due to the extra pressure behind the eyes)

At what week of pregnancy can in utero hydrocephaly often be diagnosed?

About week 16 (LMP)

How quickly will head circumference increase if rapidly expanding hydro-cephalus is present?

>2 cm/week

If a neonate is developing hydrocephalus, why should you pay attention to the *thumb* exam?

**Flexion (adduction) thumb deformity –
50 % of aqueductal stenosis patients have it**

You have just examined an apparently healthy, but macrocephalic infant. You have checked the parietal head circumference and it is large. What else should you do?

Nothing –
Unless the child develops signs of increasing ICP

A "cerebral bruit" suggests what cause of hydrocephalus?

AVM of the great vein of Galen
(The innominate vein in the chest will enlarge as a secondary effect)

How sensitive is a cranial ultrasound for detection of hydrocephalus?

98 % at 2 weeks old

How often should ultrasounds for following hydrocephalus be routinely repeated?

Every 1–2 weeks

If a cranial ultrasound suggests hydrocephalus, but your clinical exam is negative for signs of elevated ICP, what should you do?

**Serial ultrasounds –
Ultrasound findings often precede clinical findings (sometimes by weeks)**

Cranial ultrasound should be used routinely in infants less than what birthweight?

<1,500 g

If hydrocephalus is detected in utero, what is the initial management of choice?

**C-section delivery –
if the lungs are mature**

If the fetal lungs are not mature, what are the management options for hydrocephalus detected in utero?

Give steroids (for lungs) & deliver ASAP
   Or
Place shunt in utero

What medication can be useful for decreasing CSF production in hydrocephalic infants?

Acetazolamide

Hydrocephalus resulting from mechanical obstruction requires what type of treatment?

Shunting
(VP or other ventricular shunt type)

What temporary mechanical measure can be used to decrease CSF pressure in communicating hydrocephalus?

Serial lumbar punctures (LP)

What is the main objection to use of serial LPs in the treatment of communicating hydrocephalus?

1 % risk of meningitis

What is the best permanent management for most types of hydrocephalus?

Ventriculo-peritoneal shunting (VP shunting)

In general, are neurological complications decreased by early or late V-P shunting?

Early

In what age group is the risk of V-P shunt infection highest?

<6 months old

What abdominal complications can be seen with V-P shunts?

1. Organ perforation and infection introduction
2. Worsening of hydrocele
3. Worsening of inguinal hernia

What is the typical organism and timing for V-P shunt infection?

- **Staph aureus (from surgery)**
- **First 30 days**

What is the prognosis for hydrocephalic infants?

Good –
>90 % survival
(most with normal or near normal cognitive function!)

Intraventricular hemorrhage (IVH) occurring in the first 72 h of life is defined as _____?

"Early IVH"

During what postnatal period is IVH most common?

First 24 h
(50 % of cases occur in this period!)

What anatomical location do neonatal IVH's originate from?

The subependymal "germinal matrix"

When does the germinal matrix of the brain "involute," or start to disappear?

34 weeks after conception
(same as 36 weeks LMP)

Why are premature infants at such increased risk for IVH ? (2 reasons)

The germinal matrix vessels rupture easily

&

Preemies don't regulate blood pressure to the brain
(high and low system blood pressures are directly transmitted)

What is the term for the way cerebral blood flow functions in preemies?

"Pressure-passive" cerebral circulation

Why are preemies at special risk of IVH when cerebral venous pressure is high?

The germinal matrix is open to the cerebral venous system

Why do periventricular hemorrhages sometimes result in periventricular infarction?

The associated blood clot that forms may cause enough "back-pressure" to produce arterial ischemia and infarct

Is periventricular leukomalacia the same as periventricular hemorrhagic infarct?

No –
PVL is *not caused* by IVH and it is usually bilaterally symmetric (infarcts are caused by IVH and are unilateral)

Why is it a bad idea to damage your germinal matrix?

The matrix produces the neurons and glia –
Its loss may affect cortical organization, growth and myelinization

What are the main risk factors for IVH?

(3)

1. **Severe prematurity**
2. **Anything that elevates BP or causes acute BP fluctuations** (labor, seizure, abdominal exam, vigorous resuscitations)
3. **Anything that lowers O$_2$**

What is the preferred diagnostic for IVH, and what are the best alternatives?

- **Ultrasound**
- **CT or MRI**

What is the best location for ultrasound screening for IVH?
(Location with the best sensitivity)

Anterior fontanelle –
coronal & sagittal views

If you suspect a cerebellar hemorrhage, what is the best location for ultrasound screening?

Posterior fontanelle ultrasound

Infants <1,500 g require what sort of IVH screening?

US – even without symptoms

Shortly after an IVH, LP results will frequently "look like" the consequences of what procedural problem?

Traumatic LP

What percentage of LPs are *negative* in infants with *confirmed IVH*?

20 %

Persistent changes in CSF following an IVH often mimic what other important disorder?

Meningitis
(elevated protein and WBCs, decreased glucose)

LP results from neonates with IVH often mimic what three other situations/ conditions?

1. Normal
2. Traumatic tap
3. Meningitis

Elevation of what blood test suggests severe IVH has happened (or is about to happen)?

Nucleated erythrocytes

What is the relationship between indomethacin and IVH, when it is used as a tocolytic agent?

It increases IVH
(and many other bad disorders)

What is the relationship between postnatal indomethacin and IVH?

Low dose IV indomethacin decreases both incidence and severity of IVH
(*if given in first 3 days of life or so*)

Are antenatal steroids useful for IVH prevention?

Yes
(independent of effect on lung maturity)

Is vitamin K useful in prevention of IVH?

No
(although it should be given to newborns in any case)

In addition to tocolysis, what other positive effect may magnesium sulfate have on VLBW infants, when it is given antenatally?

Reduced IVH
&
Reduced cerebral palsy

In the acute phase, what are the two guiding principles in managing IVH?

Supportive care
(including correcting any bleeding risk)
&
Avoid arterial or venous pressure variation

How might UACs (umbilical artery catheters) contribute to IVH?

They produce changes in cerebral blood flow velocities when samples are taken
(or when material is infused)

In addition to indomethacin and ibuprofen, what other medication may be helpful to prevent IVH?

Magnesium Sulfate

What complications would you worry about in an infant receiving Mg sulfate?

Apnea
&
Hypotension
(at higher magnesium concentrations)

How is cerebral perfusion pressure (which is the main determinant of cerebral blood flow) calculated?

Mean arterial pressure − intracranial pressure = cerebral perfusion pressure
(MAP − ICP = CPP)

In mechanically ventilated infants at risk for IVH, what decreases risk of IVH?

Using ventilator modes that synchronize respiratory effort with machine assistance as much as possible
(reduces CBF variation)

What is the most common cause of neonatal seizures?

Perinatal asphyxia

How is the type of seizure typically seen in premature neonates suffering from perinatal asphyxia different from the type seen in full-term neonates?

- Preemies have <u>generalized</u> ***tonic*** seizures
- Term infants have multifocal ***clonic***

Mnemonic:
Tonic comes first in tonic-clonic, so younger infants have tonic, older infants have clonic. That's how you remember it

Migratory clonic seizures in the first 24 h of life are characteristic of what type of birth issue?

Asphyxia

What unusual pupillary finding is seen with asphyxia injuries in the first 24 h?

Either constriction or dilation
(constriction is worse)

In addition to perinatal asphyxia, what are three other common causes of neonatal seizures?

1. Infection
2. Intracranial hemorrhage (various types)
3. Metabolic derangements

What type of seizure usually occurs in a neonate with a subdural hemorrhage?

Focal
(The irritation is in a specific brain location)

What are the four metabolic causes of neonatal seizures you should investigate in any seizing infant?

1. **Hypoglycemia**
2. Hypocalcemia (also check Mg)
3. Hyponatremia
4. Hypernatremia

What are the usual causes of hyponatremia in a neonate?
(2)

Iatrogenic
(poor fluid management)
    Or
SIADH
(syndrome of inappropriate antidiuretic hormone secretion)

What other important electrolyte needs to be checked in any hypocalcemic neonate?

Magnesium
(If magnesium levels are not adequate, you cannot correct the calcium)

Neonates born to Moms on magnesium are prone to have what metabolic derangement?

Hypocalcemia

If a young infant is given regular cow's milk, what *metabolic derangement* may develop?

Hypocalcemia (due to high phosphorous load in the milk)

Which two groups of neonates are most likely to develop hypoglycemia?

IUGR babies (poor reserve)
&
Infants of diabetic mothers

In what three situations are you likely to see hypernatremic neonates?

1. Breast-fed neonates (inadequate fluids)
2. Iatrogenic – too much $NaHCO_3$ given
3. **Formula concentrate incorrectly diluted**

What is a rare, but very treatable, cause of neonatal seizures?
(even causes seizures in utero)

Pyridoxine deficiency

A neonate with hyperammonemia, acidosis, and neurological problems including seizures, should be checked for what metabolic disturbance?

Amino acid disorders

Three categories of recreational drug use may result in neonatal seizures. What are they?

1. ETOH
2. Opiate/opioid analgesics (heroin, methadone, etc.)
3. Sedative hypnotics

In a "mystery" newborn seizure case, what birth history question should you be sure to ask?

"Was a peripheral nerve block used?"
(on rare occasions it is accidentally injected into the fetus)

Seizures in neonates come in four categories. What are they?

1. Tonic
2. Clonic (multifocal or focal)
3. Myoclonic
4. Subtle

What are "subtle" seizures?

Those that have clear EEG findings, but are not tonic, clonic, or myoclonic

What are typical presentations of subtle seizures?

(4)

1. Eye deviation or blinking
2. Lip sucking/smacking/drooling
3. Routinized movements
   (e.g., swimming or pedaling)
4. Apnea

What patients are most likely to have subtle seizures?

Preemies

How is "convulsive apnea" different from regular (nonconvulsive) apnea?

No EEG changes
(Both are associated with bradycardia, contrary to what used to be taught)

In addition to subtle seizures, what other type of seizure is more common in premature infants?

Tonic seizures

Can tonic seizures be focal?

Yes

What types of neonatal seizures sometimes do *not* have EEG evidence of seizure?

1. Generalized tonic
2. Focal & multi-focal myoclonic

How can you differentiate myoclonic seizure activity from a jittery baby?
(3 ways)

In jittery babies:
1. Movements stop if you passively flex the area
2. Eye movements are not involved
3. Movements are in response to a stimulus (although the stimulus might not always be obvious)

In addition to getting an US, why is a head CT often helpful in neonates with seizures?

It provides much more structural information
(infarcts, calcifications, malformations, etc.)

Which two types of amino acid disorders are causes of neonatal seizure?

Maple syrup urine disease
    &
Urea cycle disorders

**What ABG finding is a clue
to the possible presence of urea cycle
disorders?**

Respiratory alkalosis
(The respiratory center is directly
stimulated by circulating ammonia)

What labs should you send to look for
amino acid disorders, if you suspect them
as a cause of neonatal seizures?
(2)

1. Urine and plasma amino acids
2. Urine reducing substances

When is the diagnostic value of an EEG
greatest for seizure disorders?

In the first few days after the first
seizure

Why is rapid intervention important
if a patient is seizing?
(2)

1. To prevent hypoxia (depending
   on type of seizure)
2. To prevent CNS damage from
   lengthy or repeated seizures

Is lorazepam (Ativan®) safe to use
in neonatal seizures?

Yes

**What are the typical first
and second-line agents for control
of neonatal seizures?**

**Phenobarbital
&
Phenytoin**

Where do most encephaloceles occur?

Occipital brain

What is an encephalocele?

Brain tissue herniated outside
the cranial cavity
(usually covered)

**What is the other name for spina
bifida?**

Myelomeningocele

What is a meningocele?

Only the meninges are outside the
vertebral column

Are myelomeningoceles generally covered
or uncovered?

Covered by meninges
(rarely covered by skin)

If a posterior vertebral arch fails to ossify
in the lower spine, is this correctly
considered to be spina bifida occulta?

Yes –
There are varying degrees of nerve
root & spinal cord involvement,
some very minimal

How does anencephaly occur?

The rostral end of the neural tube doesn't close
(leaves the cerebral tissue dysfunctional or not formed)

When is the neural tube supposed to close?

The 29th day post conception

What are the three most common neural tube defects?

1. **Spina bifida occulta**
2. **Anencephaly**
3. **Myelomeningocele**

What physical findings on the child's back may signify spina bifida occulta?
(5)

1. **Skin dimples**
2. **Very small skin defects**
3. **Hair tufts**
4. **Lipomas**
5. **Hemangiomas**

Which US ethnic group is currently at greatest risk for neural tube defects?

Hispanics

What groups(s) of mothers are generally at highest risk for having children with neural tube defects?
(2)

Low socioeconomic status
&
Extremes of maternal age
(either advanced maternal age or very young maternal age)

Pregnant women with which medical conditions are also at increased risk for neural tube defects?
(2)

Diabetes
&
Epilepsy (if taking valproate or carbamazepine)

Are neural tube defects more common in girls or boys?

Girls!
(surprisingly enough)

Which two antiseizure medications are linked to neural tube defects?

Carbamazepine (1 %)
&
Valproic acid (1–5 %)

If a person has a history of a neural tube defect, what is the probability he or she will have a child with a NTD?

4 %

What percentage of couples with children with neural tube defects has no family history of NTD?

95 %

If one child is born with a neural tube defect, what is the likelihood of having a second affected child?

About 3 %

Folic acid supplementation is very important in preventing neural tube defects. What other deficiencies contribute to neural tube defects?

Vitamin B_{12}
&
Zinc

Oversupply of this molecule (found in "hard" water, cured meat products and blighted potatoes), is also linked to neural tube defects. What is the molecule?

Nitrates

"Meckel-Gruber" syndrome consists of occipital encephalocele and what associated abnormalities?
(5 – these are the essentials for quick recognition)

1. Microcephaly/Microphthalmos
2. Polydactyly
3. Polycystic kidneys
4. Cleft lip/palate
5. Ambiguous genitalia

What specialty consultations are emergently needed for children born with encephalocele?

Neurosurgery –
The exterior tissue is often damaged and must be excised & a VP shunt is often needed

As in spinal cord injury, what part of the physical exam is especially important for the prognosis with myelo-meningocele?

**Anal tone/anal wink –
if it's present, it's called "sacral sparing," and it's is a good sign**
(Tone & presence of movement distal to the lesion level are also very important, of course!)

What special anaphylaxis risk is unusually common in infants with neural tube defects?

Latex allergy

What are the *initial management* steps for a child born with myelomeningocele, aside from the "a-b-c"s?
(4)

1. Moist sterile wrap over exposed tissues (Ask the surgeon what he/she wants – gauze is often not alright)
2. Neurosurgical consultation
3. NPO
4. IV antibiotics

In addition to performing a physical exam, what diagnostic will you want to order for infants born with myelomeningocele?

Head radiology –
US, MRI or CT
(looking for hydrocephalus or other malformations – study selected depends on surgeon, findings, previous studies)

What is the usual definitive management for myelomeningocele, and why? (2 reasons)

- **Surgical closure ≤48 h**
- **Decreases infection & prevents further loss of function**

When does hydrocephalus most commonly develop for infants with myelomeningocele?

2–3 weeks after closure

How common is it for myelomeningocele patients to have or later develop hydrocephalus?

95 % with a lumbar lesion, 2/3 with other lesions

Patients with myelomeningocele are still at high risk of death in the first year of life. What system is usually the source of their problems?

Respiratory
(apnea, aspiration, laryngeal problems)

Dysfunction of, or infection in, what organ system is a frequent cause of mortality in myelomeningocele children after age 1 year?

GU
(Neurogenic bladder leads to reflux, urosepsis, and hydronephrosis)

Delay in walking or anal sphincter control suggests that what congenital anomaly was missed?

Spina bifida occulta

Foot deformity or recurrent meningitis can be unusual presentations of what congenital neurologic abnormality?

Spina bifida occulta

How is acute renal failure defined in the neonatal period?

<0.5 cc's/kg/day

What type of renal failure is most common in neonates? (Choices are intrinsic, pre- or postrenal)

Prerenal

What is the normal urine output for a neonate?	About 2 cc/kg/h
Newborn kidneys produce unusually _____ urine. What goes in the blank?	Dilute
Radionuclide scanning is useful in cases of acute renal failure. Why?	These scans demonstrate function, not only structure (for example, DMSA & MAG-3 scans)
What dietary modification is needed for infants with renal failure?	Low protein (<2 g/kg/day)
If a neonate with renal failure develops seizures or tetany, what should you suspect first?	Hypocalcemia (If in doubt give IV calcium 40 mg/kg)
What electrolyte derangements do neonates with renal failure tend to develop?	The usual ones – high phosphate and potassium, low calcium
If a neonate has hematuria, what are the most likely causes of this uncommon problem? (3)	1. Trauma 2. Infection 3. Ischemic damage (thrombosis, asphyxia, etc.)
Neonates most commonly develop UTIs due to what organism, and by what route?	• **E. coli** • **Usually hematogenous spread**
Are girls or boys more likely to develop UTIs in infancy?	**Boys (girls get more after puberty)**
What proportion of children who develop UTIs in the first year of life has an abnormal urinary system?	**50 % (Ultrasound, VCUG, and renal scan are the basic tests)**
Barotrauma is the typical cause of air-leak syndromes (air in the chest cavity). What are some other causes to consider in neonates? (3)	1. High opening pressure when air breathing begins 2. Ball-valve gas trapping (due to mucous plug, foreign body, meconium) 3. Change in compliance with surfactant therapy

If a cross-table lateral chest X-ray reveals anterior air, or a "wind-blown spinnaker sail," what is the diagnosis?

Pneumomediastinum
(Air displacing the thymus away from the heart creates the sail)

How is pneumo-mediastinum treated?

Supportive care as needed (usually resolves spontaneously)

What is pulmonary interstitial emphysema (PIE)?

Air that has dissected into the perivascular lung tissue planes

Why does PIE cause clinical deterioration?

It produces desaturation of arterial blood, because the alveolar wall is separated from the lung capillaries (poor oxygen and carbon dioxide diffusion)

What is the X-ray appearance of PIE?

Linear radiolucencies or cystic lucencies
(may be seen throughout lung)

Although PIE has a bad prognosis, what interventions may help?

1. Decrease ventilatory pressures (inspiratory pressure, PEEP, and length of inspiration)
2. Splinting the affected side
3. High-frequency ventilation

Why is *pneumopericardium* a problem?

It acts like (is a form of) cardiac tamponade
(treat with pericardial tap/window)

In what two ways does meconium cause pulmonary problems?

Obstruction (if thick)
&
Chemical pneumonitis (irritation)

Why are infants with meconium aspiration routinely started on antibiotics?
(2)

- The X-ray appearance is the same as pneumonia
- Meconium reduces the bacteriostatic property of amniotic fluid

What is "transient tachypnea of the newborn" (TTN)?

Respiratory distress lasting <3 days in near-term or term babies

Why is TTN thought to occur?

Delayed resorption of fetal lung fluid (may also have mild lung immaturity)

**Which newborns are most likely
to develop transient tachypnea
of the newborn?**

**Term infants –
Especially after C-section**

**Does transient tachypnea of the
newborn (TTN) require treatment?**

**Generally not
(should be NPO or only orogastric
feedings, though, until tachypnea
resolves due to risk of aspiration)**

What might you be tempted to give to treat
transient tachypnea of the newborn, that
you are not supposed to give?

Diuretics
(There is sometimes fluid in the
fissures and other lung areas, but it
will go away on its own)

What chest X-ray findings are expected
in TTN?
(4)

- Prominent lung vessels
- Fluid in fissures
- Mildly flattened diaphragms
- May have pleural fluid

How are the chest X-ray findings of TTN
different from those of respiratory distress
syndrome (RDS)?

RDS is diffuse, with fluid
in the *alveoli* –
TTN is localized fluid & *alveoli are
clear*

How is transient tachypnea of the
newborn treated?

Observation, and sometimes O_2

**What is "euthyroid sick syndrome,"
and should you treat it?**
(common in premature infants)

- **Transient low thyroid
  function in association
  with a non-thyroid illness**
- **No treatment needed**

A premature neonate with low free T4
levels, but normal response to TRH,
who is not ill in any other way, has what
disorder?

Transient hypothyroxinemia
(immature thyroid –
no treatment needed)

What problems does a "vascular ring"
cause?
(2)
(*"Vascular ring" refers to the aortic arch
when it encircles the trachea & esophagus*)

Dysphagia and/or stridor
(The stridor is not usually severe)

What are the two types of imperforate anus?

High (above the muscle sling)
&
Low (may have a perineal fistula)

Do high imperforate anuses sometimes have perineal fistulas?	No
If a high imperforate anus has a fistula where will it go?	To the vagina or urinary system
How is high imperforate anus treated in the neonates?	Colostomy
How is low imperforate anus treated in the neonatal period? (two options)	Surgical perineal anoplasty Or Fistula dilation, if workable
What usually blocks the posterior nares in neonates with choanal atresia?	Bony septum (90 %) Or A membrane (10 %)
What is the best "initial management" for a newborn in respiratory distress due to choanal atresia? (2 steps)	1. Make them cry (They will breathe via mouth while crying) 2. Insert an oral airway as a temporizing measure
Incomplete separation of the larynx and esophagus, resulting in respiratory distress when trying to feed, is called…?	Laryngo-tracheal cleft
What is a fistula connecting the back of the trachea to the front of the esophagus called?	H-type tracheoesophageal fistula (3rd most common – looks like an "H" on contrast X-ray)
How is laryngomalacia usually treated, in the long-term?	**Normal growth usually eliminates the problem**
Lobar emphysema is most common in what lobes of the lung?	Upper
What *is* lobar emphysema?	Hyperexpansion of one portion of lung (compresses normal lung)
How is lobar emphysema diagnosed?	Chest X-ray
How is lobar emphysema treated?	It varies – Mild cases – observation Severe cases – resection

What pulmonary problem may mimic a diaphragmatic hernia on X-ray, but is usually easily correctable with surgery?

Cystic adenomatoid malformation

X-ray findings: Multiple separate air bubbles +/− air-fluid levels

What is cystic adenomatoid malformation of the lung?

Air-filled cysts in one or both lungs with adenomatoid tissue in at least some of them

Why do the airways of infants with congenital diaphragmatic hernias fail to develop normally?

Abnormal compression of intrathoracic contents (Both sides are affected, but defect side more than nondefect side)

What are the two main sequelae that cause problems for neonates with congenital diaphragmatic hernias?

1. Pulmonary parenchymal insufficiency (in other words, not enough lung tissue)
2. Pulmonary hypertension

What are the initial steps you should take in management of infants with congenital diaphragmatic hernias (other than the usual abc's)?

1. *Arterial line* placement (monitor blood gases)
2. *N-G* tube (decompress the stomach)
3. *Respiratory support* with "permissive hypercapnia"
4. *Surfactant* therapy (usually deficient even if full-term)

What is the most common cause of a palpable abdominal mass in a female neonate?

Simple ovarian cyst (Surgical excision is the cure – no cancer risk)

What is the most common liver malignancy in neonates, and what is its prognosis?

• Hepatoblastoma
• Bad

How is hepatoblastoma treated?

Surgical resection & follow-up chemo

In addition to hepatoblastoma, what other benign causes of liver enlargement are seen in neonates (general categories)?

(3)

1. Cysts
2. Solid tumors
3. Vascular tumors (mainly hemangioma)

When an abdominal mass is palpated in a male neonate, what is the most common source of the mass?

The kidney

What is the treatment for multicystic kidney disease detected in a neonate?

Eventual surgical resection (It is usually unilateral)

If both kidneys in a neonate have polycystic changes, what disorder are you probably dealing with, and how is it inherited?

• Infantile polycystic kidney disease
• Recessive if no family history
• Autosomal dominant if family history is positive

How does renal vein thrombosis present in a neonate?

Flank mass
&
Hematuria
(usually in the first 72 h)

What is umbilical herniation?

Abdominal contents escape through a fascial defect at the umbilicus

How are umbilical hernias treated?

They usually close in time on their own

If one or both testes are not descended in a neonate, what is the usual management?

Initially, they are observed – Many will descend spontaneously in the first few months

What is the most common cause of (congenital) obstructive uropathy in males?

Posterior urethral valves

How are posterior urethral valves managed?

Ablation of the valves is preferred (In some cases, urinary diversion is performed, instead)

Why do posterior urethral valves cause a problem?

Upstream pressure often damages the kidneys
(and they can also produce problems with continence)

What commonly performed procedure should be avoided in male neonates with hypospadias, and why?

• Circumcision!
• The tissue may be needed for later reconstruction or correction

Infants with hypospadias usually have abnormal chordee (curvature) of the penis, and often have what other abnormality?	**Cryptorchidism**
Are neonatal inguinal hernias direct, or indirect?	**Indirect**
How does a neonatal inguinal hernia or hydrocele develop?	1. **Testes pass through the processes vaginalis on the way to the scrotum** 2. **The path stays open, instead of sealing up**
When do hydroceles require surgical closure?	When they are still present at 1 year (Some clinicians consider closing them if they are still present at 6 months)
What is the appropriate management for an inguinal hernia detected in a neonate?	**Non-emergent surgical repair ASAP, if it is not incarcerated** (*5–15 % risk of incarceration in the first year* – and may be hard to diagnose rapidly)
How is a teratoma defined?	**It is a neoplasm with tissue from all three germ layers**
Where are teratomas usually found on neonates?	**Sacrococcygeal area**
How are teratomas managed?	Surgical excision
What is the other name for Wilms' tumor?	**Nephroblastoma**
Aniridia in a neonate could suggest what malignancy is also present?	**Wilms' tumor**
Why are the intestines of neonates with gastroschisis often edematous and lacking peristalsis?	The gut that is exposed is bathed in amniotic fluid – This fluid is irritating to gut (Peristalsis will spontaneously return later...)

What are the initial interventions (other than abc's) for infants with gastroschisis?

1. Temperature monitoring & regulation (big heat loss)
2. N-G decompression
3. Antibiotics (broad coverage)
4. Protective covering (as per surgery's instructions) including cellophane outer wrap to preserve heat & moisture

What is the etiology of bladder exstrophy?

The lower abdomen fails to close

What occurs in bladder exstrophy?

The posterior bladder wall sits outside the skin of the lower abdomen
(can include the whole bladder)

How is "cloacal" exstrophy different from bladder exstrophy?

It adds three components:
1. Imperforate anus
2. Omphalocele
3. Vesicointestinal fistula (often with bowel inside the bladder!)

How are bladder & cloacal exstrophy treated?

Rapid surgical repair

In esophageal atresia, what happens to the distal esophagus?

**It still forms –
In 90 % of cases it connects to the distal trachea**

Aside from inability to feed orally, what are the other main complications of esophageal atresia?
(3)

1. Bacterial pneumonia (due to atelectasis from the pressure of an air distended stomach)
2. Chemical pneumonia
3. Aspiration of saliva/feedings

What management steps are important prior to operative treatment in esophageal atresia?
(3)

1. Low intermittent suctioning of esophageal pouch
2. Respiratory support if needed
3. Broad spectrum antibiotics

What pancreatic disorder (congenital) may result in partial or total gut obstruction, and what part of the gut is affected?

• **Annular pancreas**
• **Duodenum**

How can simple (uncomplicated) malrotation cause intestinal obstruction, and what part of the gut is affected?

- **Peritoneal attachments impinge on the abnormally arranged bowel**
- **Usually duodenum**

What is "midgut volvulus," and why is it so dangerous?

- **The gut twists on its pedicle into a new orientation**
- **The superior mesenteric artery is in the pedicle! (possible loss of entire midgut!!!)**

Down syndrome, esophageal atresia, & imperforate anus are all risk factors for what duodenal disorder?

Duodenal atresia

What is the classic finding of duodenal obstruction on X-ray?

Double-bubble
(Stomach bubble & duodenal bubble are seen, then nothing else!)

How can you rule-out the surgical emergency of malrotation/volvulus in an infant with bilious emesis?

Two ways:
Upper GI
    Or
Barium enema

(If either the duodenum or the cecum is correctly positioned, it's *not* malrotation)

If the gut dies as a consequence of midgut volvulus, what parts of the bowel will be lost?

Duodenum *through ascending colon*

If a neonate has duodenal or jejunal atresia, will the abdomen appear to be distended?

No –
After all, there isn't enough gut available for the belly to get distended

What is the usual cause of jejunal atresia?

A vascular accident in utero

(damaging blood supply to that part of the gut)

"Distal" intestinal obstruction refers to obstruction in what bowel segments?

Ileum or large bowel

Other than bowel atresia, what three things might cause distal intestinal obstruction in neonates?

1. Meconium plugs
2. Meconium plug + hypoplastic left colon syndrome
3. Hirschsprung's disease

How do infants with distal intestinal obstruction present?

Same as any other patient (except that they get sick even faster)
• Distended abdomen
• Bilious emesis
• No bowel movements

What test should infants with meconium plug generally undergo?

Mucosal rectal biopsy for Hirschsprung's
(*The sweat test for* CF *is not usually diagnostic until >1 month old, and most state newborn screens evaluate for* CF *via trypsinogen levels*)

What percentage of low birth weight infants develops rickets?

30 % (!!!)

What lab finding is characteristic of rickets?

Elevated alkaline phosphatase (Calcium level is sometimes *normal*)

If you see what unusual lab result pattern, you can feel confident the diagnosis is rickets?

• **Low vitamin D**
• **Low phosphorous**
• **Low calcium**

What are the three main risk factors for development of rickets in neonates & infants?

1. Chronic disease – especially BPD
2. Very low birth weight
3. Loop diuretics

What is the typical presentation of an infant with rickets?

Poor weight gain

In severe or advanced cases of rickets, how might the infant present? (two ways)

Fractures (including ribs)
&
Respiratory distress

What is the prognosis for infants with rickets?

Excellent –
They usually recover completely

How are infants with rickets treated?	Lots of calories & Supplement calcium, vitamin D, and phosphorous
What is the relationship between the total serum calcium measured, and the ionized (active form) of calcium?	**<u>No</u> consistent relationship**
What is the *most common* presentation of hypomagnesemia?	**Hypocalcemia not corrected by calcium supplementation**
What is the usual cause of hypomagnesemia?	Inadequate intake
How does hypomagnesemia create hypocalcemia?	It decreases secretion of PTH
How is neonatal hypomagnesemia treated?	Give magnesium sulfate (IV or IM)
Why might infants with severe or chronic disease become hypocalcemic?	The catecholamines & steroids released can cause hypocalcemia (despite adequate nutrition)
A neonate requires a transfusion, then becomes hypocalcemic. Why?	EDTA or citrate (in the stored blood) complexes with calcium
Do infants (or other patients) typically experience hypocalcemia with normal volumes of blood transfusions (excluding massive or exchange transfusions)?	No
At what age is hypocalcemia most likely to develop?	First 3 days of life
What is your main concern in an *acutely* hypocalcemia infant?	**Arrhythmia**
In addition to prolonged QT & arrhythmias, what other signs of hypocalcemia may occur with a rapid drop in calcium? (2 serious, 2 less serious)	1. Seizure 2. Apnea 3. Tremor 4. Tetany

One significant source of calcium loss can be the urine. How can you measure urinary calcium losses?
(two ways)

Random spot
(compares calcium to creatinine ratio)
   Or
24-h urine

Where are the findings of bone demineralization (due to low calcium) usually seen on X-ray?
(two general areas)

Ribs & long bones

What rib finding on X-ray is typical of rickets?

"Rachitic rosary"
(Rib ends look like little balls surrounding the sternum, a little like rosary beads on a chain)

What three long bone findings are typical of rickets?

Metaphyseal:
Fraying, cupping, & lucency

How is bone demineralization typically followed over time?

Serial X-rays

Why should IV calcium be given with phosphate, when possible, when treating hypocalcemia?

If significant phosphorous isn't available, the calcium is excreted in the urine
(not in the same IV solution, though – risk of precipitation)

Why is an alkalotic infant likely to be hypocalcemic, even if his or her total serum calcium is normal?
(calcium supplementation usually needed at pH of 7.50)

The pH shift means that less of the total calcium is ionized

If alkalosis reduces the ionized calcium available in the body, what does acidosis do?

It raises it

What EKG finding is virtually pathognomonic for hypercalcemia?

Short **Q-T**

How might an infant with hypercalcemia present?
                  (4)

1. **Seizure**
2. *Polyuria*
3. **Lethargy**
4. **Poor feeding/weight gain**

Very low albumin & other serum proteins may cause what calcium disorder?	Hypercalcemia – Ionized calcium has nowhere to bind
What two medications can be used to treat hypercalcemia?	Furosemide & Calcitonin
Which medication should be used to treat hypercalcemia acutely?	Furosemide
If a patient is hypercalcemic, and also has evidence of bone demineralization on X-ray, what is the likely diagnosis?	Hyperparathyroidism
Can over-supplementation of oral calcium or vitamin D cause hypercalcemia?	Yes
A patient with hypercalcemia and osteosclerotic lesions on X-ray is likely to have what underlying diagnosis?	**Hypervitaminosis D**
What are the four likely causes of hypermagnesemia in a neonate?	1. Iatrogenic, directly to infant (of course!) 2. Mother treated with Mg sulfate (another version of iatrogenic) 3. Magnesium containing antacid given 4. Magnesium containing enema given
What are magnesium sulfate's two main effects on the body?	**CNS depressant** & **Decreases contractility of skeletal muscles**
In addition to hypercalcemia, what other cause of shortened Q-T interval might you see?	Hypermagnesemia (rare)
How is hypermagnesemia treated?	Supportive care (exchange transfusion if very severe)
How do magnesium levels get too low?	**Inadequate magnesium intake**
Can a newborn fixate visually?	Yes (about 12 inches away)

How is hypoglycemia defined in a full-term neonate?

Glucose <40

For preemies, how is hypoglycemia defined?

Glucose <40
(topic of controversy, value used can range from 30 to 50)

GE reflux, neurological, and metabolic problems can all cause neonatal apnea. Are cardiac problems known to cause apnea in neonates, too?

Yes

The group of medications used to treat apnea of prematurity, which includes caffeine & theophylline, is called _____?

Methylxanthines

Apnea of prematurity doubles the risk for what feared disorder of infancy?

SIDS
(Sudden infant death syndrome)

Does methylxanthine treatment for apnea of prematurity reduce the risk of SIDS?

No

A young infant who develops a bleeding problem after empiric treatment for rule-out sepsis has what underlying problem?

Vitamin K deficiency
(due to antibiotic wiping out the gut flora)

How much pressure is needed to open the lungs for the first breath?

20–30 mmHg

What is a normal fetal scalp pH (even if the question implies that it is not normal)?

≥7.25

What is the main reason newborns are at unusually high risk for significant heat loss?

Very high surface area compared to body mass

How is the normal heat loss of a full-term infant handled?
(3 main techniques)

• Drying
• Warm blankets
• "Radiant" warmer

Cyanosis & seizure is one of the possible presentations of what common neonatal metabolic problem?	**Hypoglycemia**
Does low glucose damage the brain?	Usually not – Prolonged seizures, and seizures with low glucose, damage it must faster
A seizure in the first 24 h of life is probably due to what problem?	Birth asphyxia
What does a neonatal seizure look like (just to review)?	Subtle – Staring, lip smacking, lack of movement, etc.
Although most neonatal seizures are due to birth asphyxia, what must you rule out first?	Metabolic and structural (hemorrhagic/developmental) causes
What are the likely neurodevelopmental consequences of neonatal seizures due to birth asphyxia?	Usually none
How are neonatal seizures treated, if they are not metabolically correctable?	Phenobarbital
Shortly after birth, a full-term neonate develops multisystem organ failure. What is the likely cause?	Birth asphyxia – It affects all of the organs, not just the brain
How is a perinatal death defined?	Death between the 28th *week* of gestation and the 28th *day* of life
How is a live birth defined?	"Expulsion or extraction" of a baby that shows evidence of life
What counts as evidence of life, in a newborn (even if the placenta is still attached)?	• Pulsating umbilical cord • Heart beat • Voluntary muscle movement
Which gender has a higher rate of infant mortality?	Males

No prenatal care increases infant mortality. What is the impact of "delayed" prenatal care?

Delay until after the first trimester correlates with higher mortality

In the US, which race has the highest infant mortality?

African Americans

The highest infant mortality is among what specific very low birth weight group, in the US?

Caucasian infants <500 g

Mortality rates for low birth weight babies have declined significantly in the past 20 years. How much improvement has occurred in low birth weight morbidity over the same period?

No significant change

What is the number one cause of infant death in the US?

Congenital malformations (about 25 %)

For *preterm* infants, what are the main risk factors for increased mortality that have to do with the baby, itself?

• Male sex
• IUGR
• Low birth weight

Which environmental problem is a common cause of increased infant mortality in the premature?

Hypothermia

Lack of which medical intervention is a risk factor for infant mortality in preterm infants?

Lack of prenatal steroids

What is the most common abnormality of the umbilicus?

Single artery

What percentage of babies with single umbilical arteries will have significant congenital anomalies?

40 %

If a newborn presents with single umbilical artery, what should you do?

Check for other congenital anomalies – Especially renal problems!

Why is placental abruption a problem?

As blood from the bleeding area organizes, it forms a barrier between the placenta and its blood supply

What is a chorioangioma, and why is it a bad thing?

Like it sounds, it's an overgrowth of fetal vessels –
If it's big, it can interfere with fetal circulation → CHF

What is the biggest risk factor for preterm delivery?

History of prior preterm delivery

What is "incompetent cervix?"

Cervical tissue that "matures" too early in pregnancy → preterm delivery

Which medication is given to prevent seizures in mothers with pre-eclampsia?

Magnesium sulfate

If premature rupture of membranes occurs (PROM), and there is also an infection, what is the best way to manage Mom and baby?

**Delivery ASAP
    &
Antibiotics ASAP
(broad spectrum)**

If PROM occurs ≥34 weeks, some obstetricians induce, while others observe for 1–2 days. From the pediatrician's perspective, what needs to be done?

**Check fetal heart rate & presentation
(either induction or observation is okay, if these look alright)**

If PROM occurs earlier than 28 weeks gestation, what is usually done? (3 things)

• **Steroids**
• **Prophylactic antibiotics**
• **Sometimes tocolysis**
   (if contractions present but no signs of infection)

Between 28 and 34 weeks gestation, what are the two options for evaluation of PROM?

1. Amniocentesis for L:S ratio to determine lung maturity
             Or
2. Steroids & bedrest until lungs are matured

Generally speaking, preeclampsia is diagnosed when abnormalities develop in what two things that are monitored during pregnancy?

Blood pressure (rising)
  &
Urine protein

What is the other name for the Group B Strep that affects neonates?

Streptococcus agalactiae
Mnemonic:
They're milk drinkers, for sure, and this bacteria puts them off their milk. "A" = without, and galactiae from the Greek root for milk (galacto like the milk sugar galactose)

For pregnant Moms with Group B Strep infection or colonization, what is the recommended antibiotic?

Penicillin
(Ampicillin is a fine alternative)

Do you need to give Group B Strep prophylaxis to a Group B positive Mom if a C-section will be done *before rupture of membranes*?

No

What is the overall idea with Group B Strep prophylaxis in pregnancy?
(popular test item!)

In general terms:
A negative culture late in pregnancy means you don't need it –
Any GBS history or risk factors means you do (*unless there is a proven negative culture late in pregnancy***)**

If a woman is about to deliver at <37 weeks, and her GBS status is not known for certain, what should you do?

Give prophylaxis

If a pregnant Mom has had ruptured membranes for 18 h or more, and her Group B Strep status is unknown, should she automatically receive Strep prophylaxis?

Yes

If a pregnant Mom is about to deliver, and she has a temperature of ≥38°, should she get Group B Strep prophylaxis?

Yes
(unless she has a known negative culture)

If a negative Group B Strep culture is obtained late in pregnancy, is prophylaxis ever needed?	No
If a Mom has a known history of Group B Strep positive results from urine, vagina, or rectum during the pregnancy, should Group B Strep prophylaxis be given?	Urine – Yes Vagina or rectum – Yes, if it was between 35 and 37 weeks *(A later negative culture means that no prophylaxis is needed)*
If a Mom has a history of a prior baby born with invasive Group B Strep, how does this affect prophylaxis?	Prophylaxis should be given *(unless there is a proven negative culture/screen)*
This Group B Strep protocol seems like a real pain. How effective has it been in decreasing early-onset Group B Strep for neonates?	70 % reduction!!! (So maybe it is worth it!)
A normal, healthy, neonate is about to be discharged from the hospital. A bagged urine specimen is reported to you with 10,000 colonies of *S. agalactiae*. What should you do? *(popular test item!)*	Nothing – It is colonization & should be left alone
What is the usual GBS prophylaxis for the Mom, if a GBS screening is positive at or near labor?	PCN IV when labor begins – Continue until labor is complete *(ampicillin or cefazolin also okay)*
What is the longest course of IV PCN given to the mother for GBS prophylaxis?	48 h (So, for example, if labor begins, then is arrested, you would still stop after 48 h even if labor isn't complete)
If Mom received GBS prophylaxis, and an apparently healthy baby is born at <35 weeks, what should you do?	Observe for 48 h (Sepsis works up if sign or symptoms of infection develop)
For infants born after 35 weeks gestation, whose Moms received GBS prophylaxis, do you need to do anything special?	Depends – If prophylaxis was more than 4 h before delivery, nothing special if needed If it was less than 4 h, *48 h of observation is needed*

What is the simplest way to screen for IUGR?

Fundal height

Reasons for an abnormally small gestational size are sometimes divided into intrinsic & extrinsic factors. How can you tell the two apart?

Intrinsic has to do with the fetus – the effect is usually general Extrinsic problems are more likely to affect only a specific area or side

If you will only have one prenatal ultrasound, when is the best time to do it?

18–20 weeks (useful for sizing/dating & also for imaging organs)

Why are ultrasounds performed after 20 weeks less useful for evaluating appropriate size and age of the pregnancy?

Rate of fetal growth is much more variable after 20 weeks

What is a level 1 ultrasound?

Just standard measurements
• Head circumference & diameter
• Femur length
• Abdominal circumference

How is a level 2 different from a level 1?

It looks at the organs & skeleton in detail

What is the "contraction" stress test?

Fetal heart rate is measured in relation to three contractions, each lasting at least 1 min

For purposes of fetal monitoring during delivery, are mothers whose labor was induced with oxytocin considered to have "high risk" fetuses?

Yes

Is a previous C-section enough to consider the fetus at "high risk" during delivery, in terms of fetal monitoring?

Yes

Are postdate fetuses considered "high risk," in terms of fetal monitoring?

Yes

If a boards vignette gives you "non-reassuring" fetal heart tracings, what is/are the correct next step(s) to take?

Fetal scalp stimulation
    &
Fetal pH monitoring
(one or both may be done)

If fetal scalp stimulation is done, what is supposed to happen?	**Fetal heart rate goes up!**
If the scalp stimulation does not produce an increase in fetal heart rate (FHR), what should you do?	**Fetal scalp pH monitor**
If fetal scalp pH is low, what should be done?	**Immediate delivery**
What is considered an abnormally low scalp pH?	**<7.2**
If fetal scalp pH is between 7.20 and 7.25, what should you do?	**Repeat in 15–30 min**
If the fetus does not respond to fetal scalp stimulation, and scalp pH cannot be obtained, how should you proceed?	**Immediate delivery based on lack of response**
What is a "saltatory" pattern of FHR?	FHR varies by more than 25 bpm, often
What is "saltatory" FHR associated with?	Acute hypoxia/ Mechanical cord compression
If Mom has a fever, and the baby's FHR is >180 beats per minute (bpm), what diagnosis should you suspect?	**Chorioamnionitis (baby's a little tachy + maternal fever)**
How would you describe a perfectly reassuring FHR tracing?	**130–150 bpm with good beat-to-beat and long-term variability**
Which should you pay more attention to – the heart rate or the beat-to-beat variability?	Variability (assuming the heart rate isn't really low)
Which fetuses are most likely to be bradycardic, as a normal variant? (2 groups)	Post-term & Transverse or occiput posterior presentations
Why does the left lobe of the liver have a higher oxygen content than the right, in the fetus?	**Blood comes to it directly after being oxygenated at the placenta (via the umbilical vein)**

What does a FHR of <80 indicate?   Very bad –
                                               Possible death soon

Do fetuses synthesize glucose?   **No!**

When do fetuses begin to store a signifi-   Near the end of the 3rd trimester
cant amount of hepatic glycogen/

What percentage of a neonate is water,   **80 %**
at the time of birth?

Roughly, what percentage of a neonate's   **Only 1/3 is extracellular**
body water is intracellular vs.
extracellular?

Normal neonates lose a significant amount   Water
of weight in the first week of life. What is   (from intracellular & interstitial
the main component of that weight loss?   stores – interesting!)

What is the target PaO$_2$ for a newborn? **About 60 mmHg**

What is the target O$_2$ saturation   **90–95 %**
for a newborn?

Is it bad to give a neonate too much   Yes
oxygen?   (various problems develop)

Is a preemie likely to be covered   **Yes –**
in vernix?   **Until about 38 weeks vernix**
                                               covers the whole baby

When does vernix first fully cover   **24 weeks**
the fetus?

Vernix is expected to be on the back,   **38–39 weeks**
scalp, and creases of the baby at what
gestational age?

At 40 weeks, how much vernix   **Just creases, mainly**
is expected?   (can be some scant vernix
                                               elsewhere)

At what age will a fetus be born without   **42 weeks!**
any **vernix?**

At what gestational age will cranial sutures no longer be mobile?	42 weeks (That could be painful!)
When will sutures still be mobile, but skull bones fully hardened?	38 weeks
The bones of the skull are very soft until what point in gestation?	27 weeks
Lanugo is different from vernix. If vernix first covers the fetus at 24 weeks, when does lanugo first cover the body?	22 weeks gestation
When does the fetus lose the fur face (lanugo disappears from face)?	33 weeks
If an infant is born at term (38–42 weeks), where do you expect to find lanugo?	Shoulders only
If a newborn has no lanugo, what is his/her gestational age?	<22 weeks or >42 weeks
Eyebrows & eyelashes appear on the fetus at what age?	23–27 weeks
Hair first appears on the fetal head at roughly what week?	Week 20 (even before the lanugo)
When will a fetus begin to lose baby hair?	Post-term (≥42 weeks)
At what gestational age does the hair tend to "stick out," with a woolly appearance, rather than lying flat?	28–36 weeks (This does sometimes come up on the exam – sorry!)
During what gestational period does the hair lie flat in pretty, silky strands?	Roughly at term (37–42 weeks) Mnemonic: The hair looks silky like baby-doll hair when they're born at the right time
Okay, enough with the hair. When do the nail plates first appear?	20 weeks (at earliest usual viability)

When do the nails reach the fingertips?	**At or near term (32–41 weeks)**
When do fingernails extend well beyond the fingertips?	**Post-term** **Mnemonic:** **Of course they're too long – they were supposed to be out to cut their nails by now!**
Very high-pitched or shrieking cries are common in which two newborn groups?	**Preemies** **&** **Neurologically impaired**
What is aplasia cutis?	**A little bit of missing skin**
Midline aplasia cutis suggests what problem?	**Spinal (or cranial) dysraphism**
Multiple areas of aplasia cutis on the scalp are what disorder's "classic presentation?"	**Trisomy 13**
A persistent posterior fontanelle + jaundice in a neonate = what disorder? Hint: Think endocrine	**Hypothyroidism**
What is Harlequin skin?	**A baby that is half pink, and half pale, divided down the midline** Mnemonic: Think of Picasso's Harlequin painting!
What is the pathological significance for Harlequin skin?	**None** **(probably autonomic variation)**
What is the earliest sign of craniosynostosis?	**Increasing bone density at the suture line**
Are neurological complications common if craniosynostosis is isolated (single suture)?	**No**
If multiple sutures are involved in cranio-synostosis, what general concept should you think of?	Congenital syndromes

How is a cephalohematoma different from caput succedaneum?

- **Cephalohematoma is a collection of blood <u>below</u> the periosteum**
- **Caput is just under the skin**

Can cephalohematomas cross suture lines?

No –
They are <u>under</u> the periosteum
(Remember that when the suture grows closed, the periosteum gets "stuck" in the sutures as they fuse. Fluids cannot cross the sutures, if they are beneath the periosteum)

Can a subgaleal hemorrhage cross suture lines?

Yes –
Blood is *under the galea* (fibrous membrane of the scalp) but *above the periosteum*

Should you do a skull X-ray following a "difficult" delivery?

No –
Not unless a significant head injury seems to have occurred (in which case CT would be better – more info)

How does subgaleal hemorrhage usually present?

A large area of scalp swelling – May *"push ears out laterally"*

Badly shaped or low-set ears are associated with many things. They are especially associated with malformation in what other organ system?

Genitourinary (GU)

In a neonate, Horner's syndrome is often due to what injury?

Lower brachial plexus injury (during the birth process)

How does Horner's syndrome present in neonates?

Ptosis Miosis & *Enophthalmos* (a little different from older children)

What effect will congenital Horner's syndrome have on the iris?

It will be lighter on that side *(Sympathetic fibers stimulate melanin production in the iris in early life)*

What is inclusion blennorrhea? | Copious discharge of mucous, that happens to have inclusions in the cells

What causes inclusion blennorrhea? | **Chlamydia trachomatis**

What causes a white pupillary reflex in a neonate?
(4 options) |
1. **Retinoblastoma**
2. **ROP**
   (retinopathy of prematurity)
3. **Retinal coloboma**
4. **Cataracts**

How are preauricular pits inherited, and how common are they? |
- **Autosomal dominant**
- **Common**

Neonates often have some nasal congestion. It can, however, be a sign of what maternal problem? | **Drug use –**
Usually opiates

Protruding tongue with a small (micrognathic) mouth, +/– cleft palate = What on the boards? | **Pierre-Robin**

What is an epithelial pearl? | **White, shiny, masses on the gum**

How are Epstein pearls different from epithelial pearls? | **Epstein pearls are found in the midline & at the hard/soft palate junctures**
(_not_ on the gums)

What is a ranula? | **A benign mass on the floor of the mouth**
(A dilated salivary gland, specifically)

Is coughing in a newborn sometimes normal? | **No –**
Frequent coughing suggests a viral pneumonia

If a neonate's chest wall moves more on one side than the other, what should that suggest to you?
(two things) |
- Intrathoracic mass
  (e.g., diaphragmatic hernia)
- Paralyzed phrenic nerve

Which heart murmurs present at birth
need to be investigated?

Those that are still there
on day 2 of life
&
Those accompanied by cyanosis,
tachypnea, or poor perfusion

**What is diastasis recti, and what is its
significance?**

- **Lack of fusion of the rectus
  muscles**
- **No significance
  (resolves spontaneously)**

**How short does the penis need
to be at birth to merit a workup?**

**<2.5 cm
(endocrine workup needed)**

**Does presence of meconium rule-out
imperforate anus?**

**No –
It can be passed via fistula**

**What is the best way to evaluate
for congenital hip dislocation?**

**Hips flexed at 90°, then abduct
until both knees are on the table –
If one or both cannot go to the
table, dislocation is possible**

Which is more likely to indicate an infant
has a syndrome – extra toes beyond the
fifth toe, or extra toes before the first toe?

Extra digits before the first toe
(same for fingers)
Mnemonic:
Makes sense – it's understandable
that you might sprout a few extra
digits in the general way they were
supposed to form. It's more abnormal
for them to form in altogether the
wrong location/direction

**When neurologically evaluating a
newborn, should flexion or extension
be greater?**

Always flexion

**Do normal-term infants have normal
deep tendon reflexes?**

Yes

Is circumcision medically indicated?

No –
Although recent studies have
indicated that it decreases heterosexual transmission of HIV

What is the finger grasp reflex?	Putting something into the baby's palm makes him/her flex and hold on
What does the baby due in the Moro reflex?	Throws its arms out with palms open
If a baby is born to a possibly infectious HepB surface antigen positive Mom, what should you do for the infant?	Clean the baby well, then: 1. Vaccinate for HepB 2. Give HepB immunoglobulin
If a neonate receives a transfusion, what screening test for the newborn may be difficult to interpret?	Hemoglobinopathy
Which three lab tests should be done shortly after birth?	Glucose Hematocrit Blood type (if Rh disease is an issue)
If a neonate's glucose is low on screen (<40 mg/dL), what should you do?	Send a serum glucose to the lab & Treat for hypoglycemia until the lab confirms the true level
How quickly should you *always* check a newborn's glucose?	Within 4 h (Sooner if there are associated risk factors for hypoglycemia: LGA, DM, SGA, very premature, maternal medications or clinical symptomatology)
If large areas of skin develop blisters or bullae on a neonate, what benign possibility should you consider?	Epidermolysis bullosa (spontaneous, or sometimes post-traumatic, shedding of the epidermis)
If a neonate develops large areas of blisters or bullae, what not benign cause should you consider?	Staph infection (!) *Emergent treatment is needed in a neonate!*
Why might O_2 requirements vary wildly in a neonate?	Sometimes the pulmonary vascular resistance varies a lot if the child has primary pulmonary hypertension (PPHN)

Better O$_2$ saturations in the upper extremities, compared to the lower extremities, is classic for what neonatal disorder? *(popular test item!)*	**PPHN**
How do the chest X-ray findings compare to the hypoxia you measure in PPHN infants?	**The hypoxia is much more extreme than you would guess from the chest X-ray**
Tachypnea with cyanosis in the first twelve hours of life is often what disorder?	**PPHN**
How often is ECMO needed in PPHN? (extra-corporeal membrane oxygenation of the blood)	5–10 % of cases
What inhaled medication has reduced the need for ECMO, in PPHN?	**Nitrous oxide**
What complication of nitrous oxide use must you watch out for? *(popular test item!)*	**Methemoglobinemia!**
In addition to nitrous oxide, what other treatment modalities are helpful with PPHN? (3)	1. Pressors 2. Sedation *without* paralysis 3. Normalization of pH, pCO$_2$, & paO$_2$ >40–60
In addition to PPHN, which other diagnoses should you especially consider for a tachypneic, cyanotic neonate (especially on the boards)? *(popular test item!)*	**TAPVR (total anomalous pulmonary venous return)** & **Underlying causes of PPHN such as polycythemia, sepsis, hypoglycemia, etc.**
What is interstitial pulmonary fibrosis?	Gradual onset of interstitial infiltrates & development of pulmonary cysts
What is the course of interstitial fibrosis?	Two options: Spontaneous recovery over months Or Cardiorespiratory failure

Which infants are most likely to develop interstitial pulmonary fibrosis?

<32 weeks & <1,500 g *without a history of hyaline membrane disease*

What are the symptoms of interstitial pulmonary fibrosis?

Slow onset of dyspnea, tachypnea, & cyanosis

What is the classic chest X-ray for interstitial pulmonary fibrosis?

Bilateral reticular infiltrates
&
**Multiple cysts
(sometimes quite large)**

A newborn with a continuous murmur & worsening respiratory status probably has what problem?
(popular test item!)

Patent ductus arteriosus (PDA)

What other physical findings are buzzwords for PDA?
(3)
(popular test item!)

- **Bounding pulses**
- **Wide pulse pressure**
- **Systolic murmur**

Would a hyperdynamic precordium go along with PDA?
(popular test item!)

**Yes –
Because the heart is working extra hard due to the unintended "recycling" of blood to the pulmonary side**

What is a hyperdynamic precordium?

The part of the chest wall in front of the heart moves much more than you would expect

If your PDA patient is ventilated, will adding PEEP improve their condition?

**Yes –
It decreases the amount of flow into the pulmonary side**

Which is more effective as a way to treat PDA, ligating the ductus or indomethacin?

They are equal

What are the main complications involved in using indomethacin to close a PDA?

- Oliguria
- Intestinal perforation
- Dilutional hyponatremia (due to too much maintenance fluid given when side effect of oliguria)

During what period is using indomethacin to close a PDA an option?

Only in the first few days of life (After that, prostaglandins are not as important, so NSAIDs don't work well)

When is indomethacin contraindicated in a neonate (4 situations)

- High creatinine or low urine output
- Bleeding diathesis or platelets <50,000
- Necrotizing enterocolitis already present
- During course of steroids

Is it alright to use indomethacin for a neonate with an intraventricular hemorrhage?

Yes

Index

A
ABO incompatibility, 70
Absence seizures, 16
Abstract reasoning, 19
Acrocyanosis, 40
ADD. *See* Attention-deficit disorder (ADD)
ADHD. *See* Attention-deficit hyperactivity disorder (ADHD)
Adrenal hyperplasia, 32
Adrenal insufficiency, 36
Alpha fetoprotein (AFP), 45
Anatomical/obstructive problems, 38
Androgen insensitivity syndrome, 32
Androgen receptors, 32
Androgens, 32
Anemia, 65, 71
Anencephaly, 108
Antenatal steroids, 60
Aortic stenosis, 63
Apgar score, 40
Aplasia cutis, 134
Apnea, 40
Apt, 38
Arthrogryposis, 83
Aspiration, 35
Association, 84
Atrial septal defects, 65
Attentional disorders, 15
Attention-deficit disorder (ADD), 14
Attention-deficit hyperactivity disorder (ADHD), 14
Automatisms, 16

B
Babble, 2
Babinski reflex, 25

Babygram, 86
Balanitis, 65
Balanoposthitis, 66
Barotrauma, 111
Beckwith's syndrome, 86
Beckwith-Wiedemann syndrome, 44, 75
Bilateral ankle clonus, 40
Bilateral cryptorchidism, 33
Biliary atresia, 39
Bili levels, 46
Bilirubin, 48
Biophysical profile, 45
Birth hypoxia, 41
Birth-related clavicle fracture, 45
Birth weight, 2
Bladder exstrophy, 118
Body surface area (BSA), 29
Body weight, 29
Bolus, 35
Botulinum, 66
Brachial plexus injury, 44
Breast abscess/mastitis, 67
Breast-fed jaundice, 47
Breast feeding, 33, 36
Breast milk, 36
Bronchopulmonary dysplasia, 58
Brown fat, 29
Bruxism, 21
BSA. *See* Body surface area (BSA)

C
Caloric requirements, 39
Caput succedaneum, 135
Cephalohematoma, 78, 135
Cerebral bruit, 99
CHARGE, 85